SECURA

AIR FRYER

COOKBOOK FOR BEGINNERS

QUICK AND EASY RECIPE FOR DELICIOUS MEALS FOR BEGINNERS

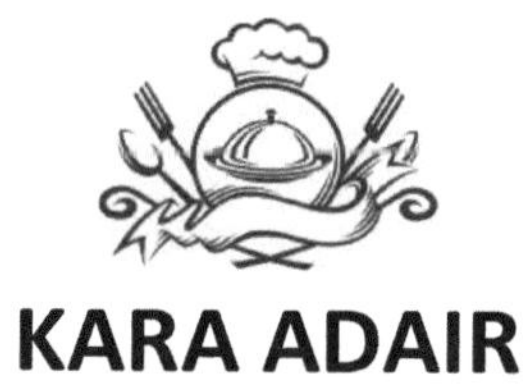

KARA ADAIR

CONTENTS

INTRODUCTION

Getting to Know Your Secura Air Fryer

An air fryer is actually a lot like a countertop convection oven. It's a small electric appliance with a heating element and a fan that blows air around in a cooking chamber. However, in an air fryer, the air is swirled very quickly in a circular fashion — so it does a better job of reaching all of the surfaces of the food and creating a crisp crust. Plus, the food itself sits in a perforated basket which increases its contact with the hot moving air. Another thing that makes a big difference? The fact that there's not much space between the walls of the chamber, and the basket intensifies the heat.

The Benefits You'll Gain from Your Secura Air Fryer

1. WEIGHT LOSS POTENTIAL

If you're driven to lose weight, you can do so by slowly making changes in your eating and cooking habits. Research shows that cooking your food with an air fryer (versus a deep fryer) can be healthier, thus potentially reducing your caloric intake and contributing to weight loss. Considering that fried food can factor into obesity, weight loss potential is among the most compelling draws of the air fryer. Additionally, the need for significantly less oil helps consumers be mindful of their cholesterol levels. Since air fryers only require a few drops of oil, it's easier to enjoy comfort food faves, like French fries, while keeping minimal saturated fat content.

2. FASTER FOOD PREP

Air fryers are very time-efficient. Foods including chicken, fish, potatoes, and vegetables all cook quickly in an air fryer. This ability is attributed to technology that allows the air fryer to blow hot air evenly within the device.

3. EASIER CLEAN UP

Not only will you exert less effort and spend less time cooking with an air fryer, but you'll also have a much easier time cleaning up. Many of its parts are designed to be wiped off with a damp cloth or washed in the sink with soap. Some air fryers even have parts that are dishwasher-safe. Overall, they're much easier to clean and maintain than larger cooking gadgets.

4. MORE SPACE, LESS STINK

Air fryers also take up less space in the kitchen, which is especially beneficial if you have a smaller space. Another bonus: An air fryer won't leave your house with lingering fried food smells for hours after cooking.

5. GREAT FOR PICKY VEGETABLE EATERS

Are you and your loved ones picky vegetable eaters? Air frying is a great way to crisp up vegetables and make them tastier. Many people enjoy the texture of vegetables such as cauliflower, broccoli, or Brussels sprouts better once they've been air fried. There are also a myriad of online recipes that give options for breading vegetables to cook in the air fryer. Some even incorporate lighter options like rice- or chickpea-based crumbs.

How You Should Start with Your Secura Air Fryer

1. PREPARATION OF THE FOOD

To prevent the food from sticking to the fryer basket, add bare minimum oil. Let space between the food to allow the hot air to pass through and cook from all sides. Use an aluminum foil paper as a separator. If you are using marinated or oily ingredients then pat them dry. This will avoid any splattering or excess smoke. Remove any oil / fat from the bottom of the fryer.

2. PREPARATION OF THE SECURA AIR FRYER

Plug in the fryer and preheat it for about 5 minutes. Ensure that your air fryer is hot enough.
Place the food items inside and avoid overcrowding. Air must be able to circulate through all the sides of each food item to properly cook it. If you are cooking pre-made foods, you can change the initial oven temperature by 70 degrees and cut the cooking time in half.

3. COOKING IN THE SECURA AIR FRYER

While cooking small food items like chicken wings or fries, try to shake the fryer around a couple of times. Also try rotating the food items every five minutes to guarantee an all-rounded fry. If you are cooking high fat food, you will find that it releases fat in the base of the fryer. You would need to remove this fat after cooking.

1. UNPLUG AND ALLOW TO COOL

After every use, unplug the air fryer from the wall outlet and allow the unit to cool completely before cleaning any component.

Wash Removable Components

Once the unit is cool, remove the crisper plate or tray and basket. These can be hand washed with dish-washing liquid and hot water or placed in the dishwasher. Always check the user guide that came with the air fryer to make sure these components are dishwasher-safe. Most manufacturers recommend hand-washing the baskets to extend their life.

2. DRY THE COMPONENTS

If you are handwashing or stop the dishwasher before the drying cycle, use a lint-free microfiber cloth to dry the crisper plate and basket. Never put damp components back into the base unit.

Wipe Down the Base Unit

Dampen a non-abrasive sponge with warm water and add a drop of dish-washing liquid. With the unit unplugged and with the basket, plates or trays removed, use the sponge to wipe out the entire interior opening. Use a microfiber cloth to thoroughly dry the area.

Rinse out the sponge and use it to wipe down the exterior of the appliance including the control panel.

3. DO A DEEP CLEAN

After several uses, check the heating element for grease splatters or food particles. Use a damp non-abrasive sponge to wipe it clean.

If the air fryer develops a bad odor, there are food splatters somewhere in the interior. In a small bowl, mix one tablespoon of water with two tablespoons of baking soda to make a paste. Dip a dampened sponge in the paste to clean the interior. You may also need to use a small soft-bristled brush like a bottle brush or an old toothbrush dipped in the solution to get into all of the corners. Rinse with a sponge dipped in clean water and dry thoroughly with a microfiber cloth before reinserting the basket and plates and plugging the unit into a wall outlet.

APPETIZERS AND SNACKS

Zucchini Fries With Roasted Garlic Aïoli

Servings: 4   Cooking Time: 12 Minutes

Ingredients:

- Roasted Garlic Aïoli:
- 1 teaspoon roasted garlic
- ½ cup mayonnaise
- 2 tablespoons olive oil
- juice of ½ lemon
- salt and pepper
- Zucchini Fries:
- ½ cup flour
- 2 eggs, beaten
- 1 cup seasoned breadcrumbs
- salt and pepper
- 1 large zucchini, cut into ½-inch sticks
- olive oil in a spray bottle, can or mister

Directions:

1. To make the aïoli, combine the roasted garlic, mayonnaise, olive oil and lemon juice in a bowl and whisk well. Season the aïoli with salt and pepper to taste.

2. Prepare the zucchini fries. Create a dredging station with three shallow dishes. Place the flour in the first shallow dish and season well with salt and freshly ground black pepper. Put the beaten eggs in the second shallow dish. In the third shallow dish, combine the breadcrumbs, salt and pepper. Dredge the zucchini sticks, coating with flour first, then dipping them into the eggs to coat, and finally tossing in breadcrumbs. Shake the dish with the breadcrumbs and pat the crumbs onto the zucchini sticks gently with your hands so they stick evenly.

3. Place the zucchini fries on a flat surface and let them sit at least 10 minutes before air-frying to let them dry out a little. Preheat the air fryer to 400°F.

4. Spray the zucchini sticks with olive oil, and place them into the air fryer basket. You can air-fry the zucchini in two layers, placing the second layer in the opposite direction to the first. Air-fry for 12 minutes turning and rotating the fries halfway through the cooking time. Spray with additional oil when you turn them over.

5. Serve zucchini fries warm with the roasted garlic aïoli.

Mozzarella En Carrozza With Puttanesca Sauce

Servings: 6   Cooking Time: 8 Minutes

Ingredients:

- Puttanesca Sauce
- 2 teaspoons olive oil
- 1 anchovy, chopped (optional)
- 2 cloves garlic, minced
- 1 (14-ounce) can petite diced tomatoes
- ½ cup chicken stock or water
- ⅓ cup Kalamata olives, chopped
- 2 tablespoons capers
- ½ teaspoon dried oregano
- ¼ teaspoon crushed red pepper flakes
- salt and freshly ground black pepper
- 1 tablespoon fresh parsley, chopped
- 8 slices of thinly sliced white bread (Pepperidge Farm®)
- 8 ounces mozzarella cheese, cut into ¼-inch slices
- ½ cup all-purpose flour
- 3 eggs, beaten
- 1½ cups seasoned panko breadcrumbs
- ½ teaspoon garlic powder
- ½ teaspoon salt
- freshly ground black pepper
- olive oil, in a spray bottle

Directions:

1. Start by making the puttanesca sauce. Heat the olive oil in a medium saucepan on the stovetop. Add the anchovies (if using, and I really think you should!) and garlic and sauté for 3 minutes, or until the anchovies have "melted" into the oil. Add the tomatoes, chicken stock, olives, capers, oregano and crushed red pepper flakes and simmer the sauce for 20 minutes. Season with salt and freshly ground black pepper and stir in the fresh parsley.

2. Cut the crusts off the slices of bread. Place four slices of the bread on a cutting board. Divide the cheese between the four slices of bread. Top the cheese with the remaining four slices of bread to make little sandwiches and cut each sandwich into 4 triangles.

3. Set up a dredging station using three shallow dishes. Place the flour in the first shallow dish, the eggs in the second dish and in the third dish, combine the panko breadcrumbs, garlic powder, salt and black pepper. Dredge each little triangle in the flour first (you might think this is redundant, but it helps to get the coating to adhere to the edges of the sandwiches) and then dip them into the egg, making sure both the sides and the edges are coated. Let the excess egg drip off and then press the triangles into the breadcrumb mixture, pressing the crumbs on with your hands so they adhere. Place the coated triangles in the freezer for 2 hours, until the cheese is frozen.

4. Preheat the air fryer to 390°F. Spray all sides of the mozzarella triangles with oil and transfer a single layer of triangles to the air fryer basket. Air-fry in batches at 390°F for 5 minutes. Turn the triangles over and air-fry for an additional 3 minutes.

5. Serve mozzarella triangles immediately with the warm puttanesca sauce.

Sweet And Salty Snack Mix

Servings: 10

Cooking Time: 12 Minutes

Ingredients:

- ½ cup honey
- 3 tablespoons butter, melted
- 1 teaspoon salt
- 2 cups sesame sticks
- 1 cup pepitas (pumpkin seeds)
- 2 cups granola
- 1 cup cashews
- 2 cups crispy corn puff cereal (Kix® or Corn Pops®)
- 2 cups mini pretzel crisps
- 1 cup dried cherries

Directions:

1. Combine the honey, butter and salt in a small bowl or measuring cup and stir until combined.

2. Combine the sesame sticks, pepitas, granola, cashews, corn puff cereal and pretzel crisps in a large bowl. Pour the honey mixture over the top and toss to combine.

3. Preheat air fryer to 370°F.

4. Air-fry the snack mix in two batches. Place half the mixture in the air fryer basket and air-fry for 12 minutes, or until the snack mix is lightly toasted. Toss the basket several times throughout the process so that the mix cooks evenly and doesn't get too dark on top.

5. Transfer the snack mix to a cookie sheet and let it cool completely. Mix in the dried cherries and store the mix in an airtight container for up to a week or two.

Buffalo Wings

Servings: 2

Cooking Time: 12 Minutes Per Batch

Ingredients:

- ➤ 2 pounds chicken wings
- ➤ 3 tablespoons butter, melted
- ➤ ¼ cup hot sauce (like Crystal® or Frank's®)
- ➤ Finishing Sauce:
- ➤ 3 tablespoons butter, melted
- ➤ ¼ cup hot sauce (like Crystal® or Frank's®)
- ➤ 1 teaspoon Worcestershire sauce

Directions:

1. Prepare the chicken wings by cutting off the wing tips and discarding (or freezing for chicken stock). Divide the drumettes from the wingettes by cutting through the joint. Place the chicken wing pieces in a large bowl.

2. Combine the melted butter and the hot sauce and stir to blend well. Pour the marinade over the chicken wings, cover and let the wings marinate for 2 hours or up to overnight in the refrigerator.

3. Preheat the air fryer to 400°F.

4. Air-fry the wings in two batches for 10 minutes per batch, shaking the basket halfway through the cooking process. When both batches are done, toss all the wings back into the basket for another 2 minutes to heat through and finish cooking.

5. While the wings are air-frying, combine the remaining 3 tablespoons of butter, ¼ cup of hot sauce and the Worcestershire sauce. Remove the wings from the air fryer, toss them in the finishing sauce and serve with some cooling blue cheese dip and celery sticks.

Cheese Wafers

Servings: 4

Cooking Time: 6 Minutes Per Batch

Ingredients:

- 4 ounces sharp Cheddar cheese, grated
- ¼ cup butter
- ½ cup flour
- ¼ teaspoon salt
- ½ cup crisp rice cereal
- oil for misting or cooking spray

Directions:

1. Cream the butter and grated cheese together. You can do it by hand, but using a stand mixer is faster and easier.

2. Sift flour and salt together. Add it to the cheese mixture and mix until well blended.

3. Stir in cereal.

4. Place dough on wax paper and shape into a long roll about 1 inch in diameter. Wrap well with the wax paper and chill for at least 4 hours.

5. When ready to cook, preheat air fryer to 360°F.

6. Cut cheese roll into ¼-inch slices.

7. Spray air fryer basket with oil or cooking spray and place slices in a single layer, close but not touching.

8. Cook for 6minutes or until golden brown. When done, place them on paper towels to cool.

9. Repeat previous step to cook remaining cheese bites.

Fiery Bacon-wrapped Dates

Servings: 16

Cooking Time: 6 Minutes

Ingredients:

- 8 Thin-cut bacon strips, halved widthwise (gluten-free, if a concern)
- 16 Medium or large Medjool dates, pitted
- 3 tablespoons (about ¾ ounce) Shredded semi-firm mozzarella
- 32 Pickled jalapeño rings

Directions:

1. Preheat the air fryer to 400°F.

2. Lay a bacon strip half on a clean, dry work surface. Split one date lengthwise without cutting through it, so that it opens like a pocket. Set it on one end of the bacon strip and open it a bit. Place 1 teaspoon of the shredded cheese and 2 pickled jalapeño rings in the date, then gently squeeze it together without fully closing it (just to hold the stuffing inside). Roll up the date in the bacon strip and set it bacon seam side down on a cutting board. Repeat this process with the remaining bacon strip halves, dates, cheese, and jalapeño rings.

3. Place the bacon-wrapped dates bacon seam side down in the basket. Air-fry undisturbed for 6 minutes, or until crisp and brown.

4. Use kitchen tongs to gently transfer the wrapped dates to a wire rack or serving platter. Cool for a few minutes before serving.

Avocado Fries With Quick Salsa Fresca

Servings: 4   Cooking Time: 6 Minutes

Ingredients:

- ½ cup flour*
- 2 teaspoons salt
- 2 eggs, lightly beaten
- 1 cup panko breadcrumbs*
- ⅛ teaspoon cayenne pepper
- ¼ teaspoon smoked paprika (optional)
- 2 large avocados, just ripe
- vegetable oil, in a spray bottle

- Quick Salsa Fresca
- 1 cup cherry tomatoes
- 1 tablespoon-sized chunk of shallot or red onion
- 2 teaspoons fresh lime juice
- 1 teaspoon chopped fresh cilantro or parsley
- salt and freshly ground black pepper

Directions:

1. Set up a dredging station with three shallow dishes. Place the flour and salt in the first shallow dish. Place the eggs into the second dish. Combine the breadcrumbs, cayenne pepper and paprika (if using) in the third dish.

2. Preheat the air fryer to 400°F.

3. Cut the avocado in half around the pit and separate the two sides. Slice the avocados into long strips while still in their skin. Run a spoon around the slices, separating them from the avocado skin. Try to keep the slices whole, but don't worry if they break – you can still coat and air-fry the pieces.

4. Coat the avocado slices by dredging them first in the flour, then the egg and then the breadcrumbs, pressing the crumbs on gently with your hands. Set the coated avocado fries on a tray and spray them on all sides with vegetable oil.

5. Air-fry the avocado fries, one layer at a time, at 400°F for 6 minutes, turning them over halfway through the cooking time and spraying lightly again if necessary. When the fries are nicely browned on all sides, season with salt and remove.

6. While the avocado fries are air-frying, make the salsa fresca by combining everything in a food processor. Pulse several times until the salsa is a chunky purée. Serve the fries warm with the salsa on the side for dipping.

Pita Chips

Servings: 4

Cooking Time: 10 Minutes

Ingredients:

- ➢ 2 rounds Pocketless pita bread
- ➢ Olive oil spray or any flavor spray you prefer, even coconut oil spray
- ➢ Up to 1 teaspoon Fine sea salt, garlic salt, onion salt, or other flavored salt

Directions:

1. Preheat the air fryer to 400°F.

2. Lightly coat the pita round(s) on both sides with olive oil spray, then lightly sprinkle each side with salt.

3. Cut each coated pita round into 8 even wedges. Lay these in the basket in as close to a single even layer as possible. Many will overlap or even be on top of each other, depending on the exact size of your machine.

4. Air-fry for 6 minutes, shaking the basket and rearranging the wedges at the 4-minute marks, until the wedges are crisp and brown. Turn them out onto a wire rack to cool a few minutes or to room temperature before digging in.

Fried Bananas

Servings: 4

Cooking Time: 8 Minutes

Ingredients:

- ½ cup panko breadcrumbs
- ½ cup sweetened coconut flakes
- ¼ cup sliced almonds
- ½ cup cornstarch
- 2 egg whites
- 1 tablespoon water
- 2 firm bananas
- oil for misting or cooking spray

Directions:

1. In food processor, combine panko, coconut, and almonds. Process to make small crumbs.
2. Place cornstarch in a shallow dish. In another shallow dish, beat together the egg whites and water until slightly foamy.
3. Preheat air fryer to 390°F.
4. Cut bananas in half crosswise. Cut each half in quarters lengthwise so you have 16 "sticks."
5. Dip banana sticks in cornstarch and tap to shake off excess. Then dip bananas in egg wash and roll in crumb mixture. Spray with oil.
6. Place bananas in air fryer basket in single layer and cook for 4minutes. If any spots have not browned, spritz with oil. Cook for 4 more minutes, until golden brown and crispy.
7. Repeat step 6 to cook remaining bananas.

POULTRY RECIPES

Chicken Rochambeau

Servings: 4   Cooking Time: 20 Minutes

Ingredients:

- 1 tablespoon butter
- 4 chicken tenders, cut in half crosswise
- salt and pepper
- ¼ cup flour
- oil for misting
- 4 slices ham, ¼- to ⅜-inches thick and large enough to cover an English muffin
- 2 English muffins, split

- Sauce
- 2 tablespoons butter
- ½ cup chopped green onions
- ½ cup chopped mushrooms
- 2 tablespoons flour
- 1 cup chicken broth
- ¼ teaspoon garlic powder
- 1½ teaspoons Worcestershire sauce

Directions:

1. Place 1 tablespoon of butter in air fryer baking pan and cook at 390°F for 2minutes to melt.
2. Sprinkle chicken tenders with salt and pepper to taste, then roll in the ¼ cup of flour.
3. Place chicken in baking pan, turning pieces to coat with melted butter.
4. Cook at 390°F for 5minutes. Turn chicken pieces over, and spray tops lightly with olive oil. Cook 5minutes longer or until juices run clear. The chicken will not brown.
5. While chicken is cooking, make the sauce: In a medium saucepan, melt the 2 tablespoons of butter.
6. Add onions and mushrooms and sauté until tender, about 3minutes.
7. Stir in the flour. Gradually add broth, stirring constantly until you have a smooth gravy.
8. Add garlic powder and Worcestershire sauce and simmer on low heat until sauce thickens, about 5minutes.
9. When chicken is cooked, remove baking pan from air fryer and set aside.
10. Place ham slices directly into air fryer basket and cook at 390°F for 5minutes or until hot and beginning to sizzle a little. Remove and set aside on top of the chicken for now.
11. Place the English muffin halves in air fryer basket and cook at 390°F for 1 minute.
12. Open air fryer and place a ham slice on top of each English muffin half. Stack 2 pieces of chicken on top of each ham slice. Cook at 390°F for 1 to 2minutes to heat through.
13. Place each English muffin stack on a serving plate and top with plenty of sauce.

Teriyaki Chicken Drumsticks

Servings: 2

Cooking Time: 17 Minutes

Ingredients:

- ➢ 2 tablespoons soy sauce*
- ➢ ¼ cup dry sherry
- ➢ 1 tablespoon brown sugar
- ➢ 2 tablespoons water
- ➢ 1 tablespoon rice wine vinegar
- ➢ 1 clove garlic, crushed
- ➢ 1-inch fresh ginger, peeled and sliced
- ➢ pinch crushed red pepper flakes
- ➢ 4 to 6 bone-in, skin-on chicken drumsticks
- ➢ 1 tablespoon cornstarch
- ➢ fresh cilantro leaves

Directions:

1. Make the marinade by combining the soy sauce, dry sherry, brown sugar, water, rice vinegar, garlic, ginger and crushed red pepper flakes. Pour the marinade over the chicken legs, cover and let the chicken marinate for 1 to 4 hours in the refrigerator.

2. Preheat the air fryer to 380°F.

3. Transfer the chicken from the marinade to the air fryer basket, transferring any extra marinade to a small saucepan. Air-fry at 380°F for 8 minutes. Flip the chicken over and continue to air-fry for another 6 minutes, watching to make sure it doesn't brown too much.

4. While the chicken is cooking, bring the reserved marinade to a simmer on the stovetop. Dissolve the cornstarch in 2 tablespoons of water and stir this into the saucepan. Bring to a boil to thicken the sauce. Remove the garlic clove and slices of ginger from the sauce and set aside.

5. When the time is up on the air fryer, brush the thickened sauce on the chicken and air-fry for 3 more minutes. Remove the chicken from the air fryer and brush with the remaining sauce.

6. Serve over rice and sprinkle the cilantro leaves on top.

Cornish Hens With Honey-lime Glaze

Servings: 2

Cooking Time: 30 Minutes

Ingredients:

- 1 Cornish game hen (1½–2 pounds)
- 1 tablespoon honey
- 1 tablespoon lime juice
- 1 teaspoon poultry seasoning
- salt and pepper
- cooking spray

Directions:

1. To split the hen into halves, cut through breast bone and down one side of the backbone.
2. Mix the honey, lime juice, and poultry seasoning together and brush or rub onto all sides of the hen. Season to taste with salt and pepper.
3. Spray air fryer basket with cooking spray and place hen halves in the basket, skin-side down.
4. Cook at 330°F for 30 minutes. Hen will be done when juices run clear when pierced at leg joint with a fork. Let hen rest for 5 to 10minutes before cutting.

Pickle Brined Fried Chicken

Servings: 4   Cooking Time: 47 Minutes

Ingredients:

- 4 bone-in, skin-on chicken legs, cut into drumsticks and thighs (about 3½ pounds)
- pickle juice from a 24-ounce jar of kosher dill pickles
- ½ cup flour
- salt and freshly ground black pepper
- 2 eggs
- 1 cup fine breadcrumbs
- 1 teaspoon salt
- 1 teaspoon freshly ground black pepper
- ½ teaspoon ground paprika
- ⅛ teaspoon ground cayenne pepper
- vegetable or canola oil in a spray bottle

Directions:

1. Place the chicken in a shallow dish and pour the pickle juice over the top. Cover and transfer the chicken to the refrigerator to brine in the pickle juice for 3 to 8 hours.

2. When you are ready to cook, remove the chicken from the refrigerator to let it come to room temperature while you set up a dredging station. Place the flour in a shallow dish and season well with salt and freshly ground black pepper. Whisk the eggs in a second shallow dish. In a third shallow dish, combine the breadcrumbs, salt, pepper, paprika and cayenne pepper.

3. Preheat the air fryer to 370°F.

4. Remove the chicken from the pickle brine and gently dry it with a clean kitchen towel. Dredge each piece of chicken in the flour, then dip it into the egg mixture, and finally press it into the breadcrumb mixture to coat all sides of the chicken. Place the breaded chicken on a plate or baking sheet and spray each piece all over with vegetable oil.

5. Air-fry the chicken in two batches. Place two chicken thighs and two drumsticks into the air fryer basket. Air-fry for 10 minutes. Then, gently turn the chicken pieces over and air-fry for another 10 minutes. Remove the chicken pieces and let them rest on plate – do not cover. Repeat with the second batch of chicken, air-frying for 20 minutes, turning the chicken over halfway through.

6. Lower the temperature of the air fryer to 340°F. Place the first batch of chicken on top of the second batch already in the basket and air-fry for an additional 7 minutes. Serve warm and enjoy.

Fiesta Chicken Plate

Servings: 4

Cooking Time: 15 Minutes

Ingredients:

- 1 pound boneless, skinless chicken breasts (2 large breasts)
- 2 tablespoons lime juice
- 1 teaspoon cumin
- ½ teaspoon salt
- ½ cup grated Pepper Jack cheese
- 1 16-ounce can refried beans
- ½ cup salsa
- 2 cups shredded lettuce
- 1 medium tomato, chopped
- 2 avocados, peeled and sliced
- 1 small onion, sliced into thin rings
- sour cream
- tortilla chips (optional)

Directions:

1. Split each chicken breast in half lengthwise.
2. Mix lime juice, cumin, and salt together and brush on all surfaces of chicken breasts.
3. Place in air fryer basket and cook at 390°F for 15 minutes, until well done.
4. Divide the cheese evenly over chicken breasts and cook for an additional minute to melt cheese.
5. While chicken is cooking, heat refried beans on stovetop or in microwave.
6. When ready to serve, divide beans among 4 plates. Place chicken breasts on top of beans and spoon salsa over. Arrange the lettuce, tomatoes, and avocados artfully on each plate and scatter with the onion rings.
7. Pass sour cream at the table and serve with tortilla chips if desired.

Parmesan Crusted Chicken Cordon Bleu

Servings: 2   Cooking Time: 14 Minutes

Ingredients:

- 2 (6-ounce) boneless, skinless chicken breasts
- salt and freshly ground black pepper
- 1 tablespoon Dijon mustard
- 4 slices Swiss cheese
- 4 slices deli-sliced ham
- ¼ cup all-purpose flour*
- 1 egg, beaten
- ¾ cup panko breadcrumbs*
- ⅓ cup grated Parmesan cheese
- olive oil, in a spray bottle

Directions:

1. Butterfly the chicken breasts. Place the chicken breast on a cutting board and press down on the breast with the palm of your hand. Slice into the long side of the chicken breast, parallel to the cutting board, but not all the way through to the other side. Open the chicken breast like a "book". Place a piece of plastic wrap over the chicken breast and gently pound it with a meat mallet to make it evenly thick.

2. Season the chicken with salt and pepper. Spread the Dijon mustard on the inside of each chicken breast. Layer one slice of cheese on top of the mustard, then top with the 2 slices of ham and the other slice of cheese.

3. Starting with the long edge of the chicken breast, roll the chicken up to the other side. Secure it shut with 1 or 2 toothpicks.

4. Preheat the air fryer to 350°F.

5. Set up a dredging station with three shallow dishes. Place the flour in the first dish. Place the beaten egg in the second shallow dish. Combine the panko breadcrumbs and Parmesan cheese together in the third shallow dish. Dip the stuffed and rolled chicken breasts in the flour, then the beaten egg and then roll in the breadcrumb-cheese mixture to cover on all sides. Press the crumbs onto the chicken breasts with your hands to make sure they are well adhered. Spray the chicken breasts with olive oil and transfer to the air fryer basket.

6. Air-fry at 350°F for 14 minutes, flipping the breasts over halfway through the cooking time. Let the chicken rest for a few minutes before removing the toothpicks, slicing and serving.

Gluten-free Nutty Chicken Fingers

Servings: 4

Cooking Time: 10 Minutes

Ingredients:

- ½ cup gluten-free flour
- ½ teaspoon garlic powder
- ¼ teaspoon onion powder
- ¼ teaspoon black pepper
- ¼ teaspoon salt
- 1 cup walnuts, pulsed into coarse flour
- ½ cup gluten-free breadcrumbs
- 2 large eggs
- 1 pound boneless, skinless chicken tenders

Directions:

1. Preheat the air fryer to 400°F.
2. In a medium bowl, mix the flour, garlic, onion, pepper, and salt. Set aside.
3. In a separate bowl, mix the walnut flour and breadcrumbs.
4. In a third bowl, whisk the eggs.
5. Liberally spray the air fryer basket with olive oil spray.
6. Pat the chicken tenders dry with a paper towel. Dredge the tenders one at a time in the flour, then dip them in the egg, and toss them in the breadcrumb coating. Repeat until all tenders are coated.
7. Set each tender in the air fryer, leaving room on each side of the tender to allow for flipping.
8. When the basket is full, cook 5 minutes, flip, and cook another 5 minutes. Check the internal temperature after cooking completes; it should read 165°F. If it does not, cook another 2 to 4 minutes.
9. Remove the tenders and let cool 5 minutes before serving. Repeat until all the tenders are cooked.

Coconut Curry Chicken With Coconut Rice

Servings: 4   Cooking Time: 56 Minutes

Ingredients:

- 1 (14-ounce) can coconut milk
- 2 tablespoons green or red curry paste
- zest and juice of one lime
- 1 clove garlic, minced
- 1 tablespoon grated fresh ginger
- 1 teaspoon ground cumin
- 1 (3- to 4-pound) chicken, cut into 8 pieces
- vegetable or olive oil
- salt and freshly ground black pepper
- fresh cilantro leaves
- For the rice:
- 1 cup basmati or jasmine rice
- 1 cup water
- 1 cup coconut milk
- ½ teaspoon salt
- freshly ground black pepper

Directions:

1. Make the marinade by combining the coconut milk, curry paste, lime zest and juice, garlic, ginger and cumin. Coat the chicken on all sides with the marinade and marinate the chicken for 1 hour to overnight in the refrigerator.

2. Preheat the air fryer to 380°F.

3. Brush the bottom of the air fryer basket with oil. Transfer the chicken thighs and drumsticks from the marinade to the air fryer basket, letting most of the marinade drip off. Season to taste with salt and freshly ground black pepper.

4. Air-fry the chicken drumsticks and thighs at 380°F for 12 minutes. Flip the chicken over and continue to air-fry for another 12 minutes. Set aside and air-fry the chicken breast pieces at 380°F for 15 minutes. Turn the chicken breast pieces over and air-fry for another 12 minutes. Return the chicken thighs and drumsticks to the air fryer and air-fry for an additional 5 minutes.

5. While the chicken is cooking, make the coconut rice. Rinse the rice kernels with water and drain well. Place the rice in a medium saucepan with a tight fitting lid, along with the water, coconut milk, salt and freshly ground black pepper. Bring the mixture to a boil and then cover, reduce the heat and let it cook gently for 20 minutes without lifting the lid. When the time is up, lift the lid, fluff with a fork and set aside.

6. Remove the chicken from the air fryer and serve warm with the coconut rice and fresh cilantro scattered around.

Thai Chicken Drumsticks

Servings: 4

Cooking Time: 20 Minutes

Ingredients:

- 2 tablespoons soy sauce
- ¼ cup rice wine vinegar
- 2 tablespoons chili garlic sauce
- 2 tablespoons sesame oil
- 1 teaspoon minced fresh ginger
- 2 teaspoons sugar
- ½ teaspoon ground coriander
- juice of 1 lime
- 8 chicken drumsticks (about 2½ pounds)
- ¼ cup chopped peanuts
- chopped fresh cilantro
- lime wedges

Directions:

1. Combine the soy sauce, rice wine vinegar, chili sauce, sesame oil, ginger, sugar, coriander and lime juice in a large bowl and mix together. Add the chicken drumsticks and marinate for 30 minutes.

2. Preheat the air fryer to 370°F.

3. Place the chicken in the air fryer basket. It's ok if the ends of the drumsticks overlap a little. Spoon half of the marinade over the chicken, and reserve the other half.

4. Air-fry for 10 minutes. Turn the chicken over and pour the rest of the marinade over the chicken. Air-fry for an additional 10 minutes.

5. Transfer the chicken to a plate to rest and cool to an edible temperature. Pour the marinade from the bottom of the air fryer into a small saucepan and bring it to a simmer over medium-high heat. Simmer the liquid for 2 minutes so that it thickens enough to coat the back of a spoon.

6. Transfer the chicken to a serving platter, pour the sauce over the chicken and sprinkle the chopped peanuts on top. Garnish with chopped cilantro and lime wedges.

Southern-fried Chicken Livers

Servings: 4

Cooking Time: 12 Minutes

Ingredients:

- 2 eggs
- 2 tablespoons water
- ¾ cup flour
- 1½ cups panko breadcrumbs
- ½ cup plain breadcrumbs
- 1 teaspoon salt
- ½ teaspoon black pepper
- 20 ounces chicken livers, salted to taste
- oil for misting or cooking spray

Directions:

1. Beat together eggs and water in a shallow dish. Place the flour in a separate shallow dish.

2. In the bowl of a food processor, combine the panko, plain breadcrumbs, salt, and pepper. Process until well mixed and panko crumbs are finely crushed. Place crumbs in a third shallow dish.

3. Dip livers in flour, then egg wash, and then roll in panko mixture to coat well with crumbs.

4. Spray both sides of livers with oil or cooking spray. Cooking in two batches, place livers in air fryer basket in single layer.

5. Cook at 390°F for 7minutes. Spray livers, turn over, and spray again. Cook for 5 more minutes, until done inside and coating is golden brown.

6. Repeat to cook remaining livers.

BEEF , PORK & LAMB RECIPES

Glazed Meatloaf

Servings: 4   Cooking Time: 35-55 Minutes

Ingredients:

- ½ cup Seasoned Italian-style panko bread crumbs (gluten-free, if a concern)
- ¼ cup Whole or low-fat milk
- 1 pound Lean ground beef
- 1 pound Bulk mild Italian sausage meat (gluten-free, if a concern)
- 1 Large egg(s), well beaten
- 1 teaspoon Dried thyme
- 1 teaspoon Onion powder
- 1 teaspoon Garlic powder
- Vegetable oil spray
- 1 tablespoon Ketchup (gluten-free, if a concern)
- 1 tablespoon Hoisin sauce (see here; gluten-free, if a concern)
- 2 teaspoons Pickle brine, preferably from a jar of jalapeño rings (gluten-free, if a concern)

Directions:

1. Pour the bread crumbs into a large bowl, add the milk, stir gently, and soak for 10 minutes.

2. Preheat the air fryer to 350°F .

3. Add the ground beef, Italian sausage meat, egg(s), thyme, onion powder, and garlic powder to the bowl with the bread crumbs. Blend gently until well combined. (Clean, dry hands work best!) Form this mixture into an oval loaf about 2 inches tall (its length will vary depending on the amount of ingredients) but with a flat bottom. Generously coat the top, bottom, and all sides of the loaf with vegetable oil spray.

4. Use a large, nonstick-safe spatula or perhaps silicone baking mitts to transfer the loaf to the basket. Air-fry undisturbed for 30 minutes for a small meatloaf, 40 minutes for a medium one, or 50 minutes for a large, until an instant-read meat thermometer inserted into the center of the loaf registers 165°F.

5. Whisk the ketchup, hoisin, and pickle brine in a small bowl until smooth. Brush this over the top and sides of the meatloaf and continue air-frying undisturbed for 5 minutes, or until the glaze has browned a bit. Use that same spatula or those same baking mitts to transfer the meatloaf to a cutting board. Cool for 10 minutes before slicing.

T-bone Steak With Roasted Tomato, Corn And Asparagus Salsa

Servings: 2

Cooking Time: 15-20 Minutes

Ingredients:

- 1 (20-ounce) T-bone steak
- salt and freshly ground black pepper
- Salsa
- 1½ cups cherry tomatoes
- ¾ cup corn kernels (fresh, or frozen and thawed)
- 1½ cups sliced asparagus (1-inch slices) (about ½ bunch)
- 1 tablespoon + 1 teaspoon olive oil, divided
- salt and freshly ground black pepper
- 1½ teaspoons red wine vinegar
- 3 tablespoons chopped fresh basil
- 1 tablespoon chopped fresh chives

Directions:

1. Preheat the air fryer to 400°F.

2. Season the steak with salt and pepper and air-fry at 400°F for 10 minutes (medium-rare), 12 minutes (medium), or 15 minutes (well-done), flipping the steak once halfway through the cooking time.

3. In the meantime, toss the tomatoes, corn and asparagus in a bowl with a teaspoon or so of olive oil, salt and freshly ground black pepper.

4. When the steak has finished cooking, remove it to a cutting board, tent loosely with foil and let it rest. Transfer the vegetables to the air fryer and air-fry at 400°F for 5 minutes, shaking the basket once or twice during the cooking process. Transfer the cooked vegetables back into the bowl and toss with the red wine vinegar, remaining olive oil and fresh herbs.

5. To serve, slice the steak on the bias and serve with some of the salsa on top.

Spicy Hoisin Bbq Pork Chops

Servings: 2

Cooking Time: 12 Minutes

Ingredients:

➢ 3 tablespoons hoisin sauce

➢ ¼ cup honey

➢ 1 tablespoon soy sauce

➢ 3 tablespoons rice vinegar

➢ 2 tablespoons brown sugar

➢ 1½ teaspoons grated fresh ginger

➢ 1 to 2 teaspoons Sriracha sauce, to taste

➢ 2 to 3 bone-in center cut pork chops, 1-inch thick (about 1¼ pounds)

➢ chopped scallions, for garnish

Directions:

1. Combine the hoisin sauce, honey, soy sauce, rice vinegar, brown sugar, ginger, and Sriracha sauce in a small saucepan. Whisk the ingredients together and bring the mixture to a boil over medium-high heat on the stovetop. Reduce the heat and simmer the sauce until it has reduced in volume and thickened slightly – about 10 minutes.

2. Preheat the air fryer to 400°F.

3. Place the pork chops into the air fryer basket and pour half the hoisin BBQ sauce over the top. Air-fry for 6 minutes. Then, flip the chops over, pour the remaining hoisin BBQ sauce on top and air-fry for 6 more minutes, depending on the thickness of the pork chops. The internal temperature of the pork chops should be 155°F when tested with an instant read thermometer.

4. Let the pork chops rest for 5 minutes before serving. You can spoon a little of the sauce from the bottom drawer of the air fryer over the top if desired. Sprinkle with chopped scallions and serve.

Bourbon Bacon Burgers

| Servings: 2 | Cooking Time: 23-28 Minutes |

Ingredients:

- 1 tablespoon bourbon
- 2 tablespoons brown sugar
- 3 strips maple bacon, cut in half
- ¾ pound ground beef (80% lean)
- 1 tablespoon minced onion
- 2 tablespoons BBQ sauce
- ½ teaspoon salt
- freshly ground black pepper
- 2 slices Colby Jack cheese (or Monterey Jack)
- 2 Kaiser rolls
- lettuce and tomato, for serving
- Zesty Burger Sauce:
- 2 tablespoons BBQ sauce
- 2 tablespoons mayonnaise
- ¼ teaspoon ground paprika
- freshly ground black pepper

Directions:

1. Preheat the air fryer to 390°F and pour a little water into the bottom of the air fryer drawer. (This will help prevent the grease that drips into the bottom drawer from burning and smoking.)

2. Combine the bourbon and brown sugar in a small bowl. Place the bacon strips in the air fryer basket and brush with the brown sugar mixture. Air-fry at 390°F for 4 minutes. Flip the bacon over, brush with more brown sugar and air-fry at 390°F for an additional 4 minutes until crispy.

3. While the bacon is cooking, make the burger patties. Combine the ground beef, onion, BBQ sauce, salt and pepper in a large bowl. Mix together thoroughly with your hands and shape the meat into 2 patties.

4. Transfer the burger patties to the air fryer basket and air-fry the burgers at 370°F for 15 to 20 minutes, depending on how you like your burger cooked (15 minutes for rare to medium-rare; 20 minutes for well-done). Flip the burgers over halfway through the cooking process.

5. While the burgers are air-frying, make the burger sauce by combining the BBQ sauce, mayonnaise, paprika and freshly ground black pepper in a bowl.

6. When the burgers are cooked to your liking, top each patty with a slice of Colby Jack cheese and air-fry for an additional minute, just to melt the cheese. (You might want to pin the cheese slice to the burger with a toothpick to prevent it from blowing off in your air fryer.) Spread the sauce on the inside of the Kaiser rolls, place the burgers on the rolls, top with the bourbon bacon, lettuce and tomato and enjoy!

Pork Schnitzel With Dill Sauce

Servings: 4

Cooking Time: 4 Minutes

Ingredients:

- 6 boneless, center cut pork chops (about 1½ pounds)
- ½ cup flour
- 1½ teaspoons salt
- freshly ground black pepper
- 2 eggs
- ½ cup milk
- 1½ cups toasted fine breadcrumbs
- 1 teaspoon paprika
- 3 tablespoons butter, melted
- 2 tablespoons vegetable or olive oil
- lemon wedges
- Dill Sauce:
- 1 cup chicken stock
- 1½ tablespoons cornstarch
- ⅓ cup sour cream
- 1½ tablespoons chopped fresh dill
- salt and pepper

Directions:

1. Trim the excess fat from the pork chops and pound each chop with a meat mallet between two pieces of plastic wrap until they are ½-inch thick.

2. Set up a dredging station. Combine the flour, salt, and black pepper in a shallow dish. Whisk the eggs and milk together in a second shallow dish. Finally, combine the breadcrumbs and paprika in a third shallow dish.

3. Dip each flattened pork chop in the flour. Shake off the excess flour and dip each chop into the egg mixture. Finally dip them into the breadcrumbs and press the breadcrumbs onto the meat firmly. Place each finished chop on a baking sheet until they are all coated.

4. Preheat the air fryer to 400°F.

5. Combine the melted butter and the oil in a small bowl and lightly brush both sides of the coated pork chops. Do not brush the chops too heavily or the breading will not be as crispy.

6. Air-fry one schnitzel at a time for 4 minutes, turning it over halfway through the cooking time. Hold the cooked schnitzels warm on a baking pan in a 170°F oven while you finish air-frying the rest.

7. While the schnitzels are cooking, whisk the chicken stock and cornstarch together in a small saucepan over medium-high heat on the stovetop. Bring the mixture to a boil and simmer for 2 minutes. Remove the saucepan from heat and whisk in the sour cream. Add the chopped fresh dill and season with salt and pepper.

8. Transfer the pork schnitzel to a platter and serve with dill sauce and lemon wedges. For a traditional meal, serve this along side some egg noodles, spätzle or German potato salad.

Bacon Wrapped Filets Mignons

Servings: 4

Cooking Time: 18 Minutes

Ingredients:

- ➤ 4 slices bacon (not thick cut)
- ➤ 4 (8-ounce) filets mignons
- ➤ 1 tablespoon fresh thyme leaves
- ➤ salt and freshly ground black pepper

Directions:

1. Preheat the air fryer to 400°F.

2. Lay the bacon slices down on a cutting board and sprinkle the thyme leaves on the bacon slices. Remove any string tying the filets and place the steaks down on their sides on top of the bacon slices. Roll the bacon around the side of the filets and secure the bacon to the fillets with a toothpick or two.

3. Season the steaks generously with salt and freshly ground black pepper and transfer the steaks to the air fryer.

4. Air-fry for 18 minutes, turning the steaks over halfway through the cooking process. This should cook your steaks to about medium, depending on how thick they are. If you'd prefer your steaks medium-rare or medium-well, simply add or subtract two minutes from the cooking time. Remove the steaks from the air fryer and let them rest for 5 minutes before removing the toothpicks and serving. (Just enough time to quickly air-fry some vegetables to go with them!)

Pork & Beef Egg Rolls

Servings: 8

Cooking Time: 8 Minutes

Ingredients:

- ¼ pound very lean ground beef
- ¼ pound lean ground pork
- 1 tablespoon soy sauce
- 1 teaspoon olive oil
- ½ cup grated carrots
- 2 green onions, chopped
- 2 cups grated Napa cabbage
- ¼ cup chopped water chestnuts
- ¼ teaspoon salt
- ¼ teaspoon garlic powder
- ¼ teaspoon black pepper
- 1 egg
- 1 tablespoon water
- 8 egg roll wraps
- oil for misting or cooking spray

Directions:

1. In a large skillet, brown beef and pork with soy sauce. Remove cooked meat from skillet, drain, and set aside.

2. Pour off any excess grease from skillet. Add olive oil, carrots, and onions. Sauté until barely tender, about 1 minute.

3. Stir in cabbage, cover, and cook for 1 minute or just until cabbage slightly wilts. Remove from heat.

4. In a large bowl, combine the cooked meats and vegetables, water chestnuts, salt, garlic powder, and pepper. Stir well. If needed, add more salt to taste.

5. Beat together egg and water in a small bowl.

6. Fill egg roll wrappers, using about ¼ cup of filling for each wrap. Roll up and brush all over with egg wash to seal. Spray very lightly with olive oil or cooking spray.

7. Place 4 egg rolls in air fryer basket and cook at 390°F for 4minutes. Turn over and cook 4 more minutes, until golden brown and crispy.

8. Repeat to cook remaining egg rolls.

Kielbasa Sausage With Pierogies And Caramelized Onions

Servings: 3

Cooking Time: 30 Minutes

Ingredients:

- 1 Vidalia or sweet onion, sliced
- olive oil
- salt and freshly ground black pepper
- 2 tablespoons butter, cut into small cubes
- 1 teaspoon sugar
- 1 pound light Polish kielbasa sausage, cut into 2-inch chunks
- 1 (13-ounce) package frozen mini pierogies
- 2 teaspoons vegetable or olive oil
- chopped scallions

Directions:

1. Preheat the air fryer to 400°F.

2. Toss the sliced onions with a little olive oil, salt and pepper and transfer them to the air fryer basket. Dot the onions with pieces of butter and air-fry at 400°F for 2 minutes. Then sprinkle the sugar over the onions and stir. Pour any melted butter from the bottom of the air fryer drawer over the onions (do this over the sink – some of the butter will spill through the basket). Continue to air-fry for another 13 minutes, stirring or shaking the basket every few minutes to cook the onions evenly.

3. Add the kielbasa chunks to the onions and toss. Air-fry for another 5 minutes, shaking the basket halfway through the cooking time. Transfer the kielbasa and onions to a bowl and cover with aluminum foil to keep warm.

4. Toss the frozen pierogies with the vegetable or olive oil and transfer them to the air fryer basket. Air-fry at 400°F for 8 minutes, shaking the basket twice during the cooking time.

5. When the pierogies have finished cooking, return the kielbasa and onions to the air fryer and gently toss with the pierogies. Air-fry for 2 more minutes and then transfer everything to a serving platter. Garnish with the chopped scallions and serve hot with the spicy sour cream sauce below.

6. Kielbasa Sausage with Pierogies and Caramelized Onions

Pork Loin

Servings: 8

Cooking Time: 50 Minutes

Ingredients:

- ➢ 1 tablespoon lime juice
- ➢ 1 tablespoon orange marmalade
- ➢ 1 teaspoon coarse brown mustard
- ➢ 1 teaspoon curry powder
- ➢ 1 teaspoon dried lemongrass
- ➢ 2-pound boneless pork loin roast
- ➢ salt and pepper
- ➢ cooking spray

Directions:

1. Mix together the lime juice, marmalade, mustard, curry powder, and lemongrass.
2. Rub mixture all over the surface of the pork loin. Season to taste with salt and pepper.
3. Spray air fryer basket with nonstick spray and place pork roast diagonally in basket.
4. Cook at 360°F for approximately 50 minutes, until roast registers 130°F on a meat thermometer.
5. Wrap roast in foil and let rest for 10minutes before slicing.

Korean-style Lamb Shoulder Chops

Servings: 3

Cooking Time: 28 Minutes

Ingredients:

➢ ⅓ cup Regular or low-sodium soy sauce or gluten-free tamari sauce

➢ 1½ tablespoons Toasted sesame oil

➢ 1½ tablespoons Granulated white sugar

➢ 2 teaspoons Minced peeled fresh ginger

➢ 1 teaspoon Minced garlic

➢ ¼ teaspoon Red pepper flakes

➢ 3 6-ounce bone-in lamb shoulder chops, any excess fat trimmed

➢ ⅔ cup Tapioca flour

➢ Vegetable oil spray

Directions:

1. Put the soy or tamari sauce, sesame oil, sugar, ginger, garlic, and red pepper flakes in a large, heavy zip-closed plastic bag. Add the chops, seal, and rub the marinade evenly over them through the bag. Refrigerate for at least 2 hours or up to 6 hours, turning the bag at least once so the chops move around in the marinade.

2. Set the bag out on the counter as the air fryer heats. Preheat the air fryer to 375°F .

3. Pour the tapioca flour on a dinner plate or in a small pie plate. Remove a chop from the marinade and dredge it on both sides in the tapioca flour, coating it evenly and well. Coat both sides with vegetable oil spray, set it in the basket, and dredge and spray the remaining chop(s), setting them in the basket in a single layer with space between them. Discard the bag with the marinade.

4. Air-fry, turning once, for 25 minutes, or until the chops are well browned and tender when pierced with the point of a paring knife. If the machine is at 360°F, you may need to add up to 3 minutes to the cooking time.

5. Use kitchen tongs to transfer the chops to a wire rack. Cool for just a couple of minutes before serving.

Rack Of Lamb With Pistachio Crust

Servings: 2

Cooking Time: 19 Minutes

Ingredients:

- ½ cup finely chopped pistachios
- 3 tablespoons panko breadcrumbs
- 1 teaspoon chopped fresh rosemary
- 2 teaspoons chopped fresh oregano
- salt and freshly ground black pepper
- 1 tablespoon olive oil
- 1 rack of lamb, bones trimmed of fat and frenched
- 1 tablespoon Dijon mustard

Directions:

1. Preheat the air fryer to 380°F.

2. Combine the pistachios, breadcrumbs, rosemary, oregano, salt and pepper in a small bowl. Drizzle in the olive oil and stir to combine.

3. Season the rack of lamb with salt and pepper on all sides and transfer it to the air fryer basket with the fat side facing up. Air-fry the lamb for 12 minutes. Remove the lamb from the air fryer and brush the fat side of the lamb rack with the Dijon mustard. Coat the rack with the pistachio mixture, pressing the breadcrumbs onto the lamb with your hands and rolling the bottom of the rack in any of the crumbs that fall off.

4. Return the rack of lamb to the air fryer and air-fry for another 3 to 7 minutes or until an instant read thermometer reads 140°F for medium. Add or subtract a couple of minutes for lamb that is more or less well cooked. (Your time will vary depending on how big the rack of lamb is.)

5. Let the lamb rest for at least 5 minutes. Then, slice into chops and serve.

Garlic And Oregano Lamb Chops

Servings: 4

Cooking Time: 17 Minutes

Ingredients:

- 1½ tablespoons Olive oil
- 1 tablespoon Minced garlic
- 1 teaspoon Dried oregano
- 1 teaspoon Finely minced orange zest
- ¾ teaspoon Fennel seeds
- ¾ teaspoon Table salt
- ¾ teaspoon Ground black pepper
- 6 4-ounce, 1-inch-thick lamb loin chops

Directions:

1. Mix the olive oil, garlic, oregano, orange zest, fennel seeds, salt, and pepper in a large bowl. Add the chops and toss well to coat. Set aside as the air fryer heats, tossing one more time.

2. Preheat the air fryer to 400°F.

3. Set the chops bone side down in the basket (that is, so they stand up on their bony edge) with as much air space between them as possible. Air-fry undisturbed for 14 minutes for medium-rare, or until an instant-read meat thermometer inserted into the thickest part of a chop (without touching bone) registers 132°F (not USDA-approved). Or air-fry undisturbed for 17 minutes for well done, or until an instant-read meat thermometer registers 145°F (USDA-approved).

4. Use kitchen tongs to transfer the chops to a wire rack. Cool for 5 minutes before serving.

VEGETABLE SIDE DISHES RECIPES

Tomato Candy

Servings: 12

Cooking Time: 120 Minutes

Ingredients:

- ➢ 6 Small Roma or plum tomatoes, halved lengthwise
- ➢ 1½ teaspoons Coarse sea salt or kosher salt

Directions:

1. Before you turn the machine on, set the tomatoes cut side up in a single layer in the basket (or the basket attachment). They can touch each other, but try to leave at least a fraction of an inch between them (depending, of course, on the size of the basket or basket attachment). Sprinkle the cut sides of the tomatoes with the salt.

2. Set the machine to cook at 225°F (or 230°F, if that's the closest setting). Put the basket in the machine and air-fry for 2 hours, or until the tomatoes are dry but pliable, with a little moisture down in their centers.

3. Remove the basket from the machine and cool the tomatoes in it for 10 minutes before gently transferring them to a plate for serving, or to a shallow dish that you can cover and store in the refrigerator for up to 1 week.

Steak Fries

Cooking Time: 20 Minutes

Servings: 4

Ingredients:

- ➤ 2 russet potatoes, scrubbed and cut into wedges lengthwise
- ➤ 1 tablespoon olive oil
- ➤ 2 teaspoons seasoning salt (recipe below)

Directions:

1. Preheat the air fryer to 400°F.
2. Toss the potatoes with the olive oil and the seasoning salt.
3. Air-fry for 20 minutes (depending on the size of the wedges), turning the potatoes over gently a few times throughout the cooking process to brown and cook them evenly.

General Tso's Cauliflower

Servings: 3   Cooking Time: 15 Minutes

Ingredients:

- ⅓ cup All-purpose flour or tapioca flour
- 2 Large egg(s), well beaten
- ⅔ cup Plain panko bread crumbs (gluten-free, if a concern)
- 2½ cups (about 13 ounces) 1½-inch cauliflower florets
- Vegetable oil spray
- 2 tablespoons Regular or low-sodium soy sauce or gluten-free tamari sauce
- 1 tablespoon Hoisin sauce (gluten-free, if a concern; see here)
- 1 tablespoon Unseasoned rice vinegar (see here)
- 2 teaspoons Granulated white sugar
- 1½ teaspoons Sriracha or other hot red pepper sauce (gluten-free, if a concern)
- Not needed Water
- Not needed Cornstarch

Directions:

1. Preheat the air fryer to 400°F.

2. Put the flour in one zip-closed plastic bag, the beaten egg in a second bag, and the bread crumbs in a third.

3. Put the cauliflower florets in the bag with the flour. Seal closed, then shake and turn to coat the florets completely. Open the bag and transfer the florets to the bag with the egg(s). (Do not just dump the florets from one bag into the other.) Seal the second bag and turn gently to coat the florets in the egg(s). Open the second bag and use kitchen tongs to transfer the florets to the third bag. Seal that bag; shake and turn it to coat the florets in the bread crumbs.

4. Spread paper towels on your work surface. Gently transfer the florets to these paper towels, then coat them with vegetable oil spray on all sides.

5. Gently spread the florets in the basket in as close to one layer as you can. Air-fry undisturbed for 15 minutes, or until crisp and browned.

6. Meanwhile, stir the soy sauce or tamari sauce, hoisin sauce, vinegar, sugar, and sriracha in a small saucepan set over medium heat until smooth. Bring to a simmer, stirring often. Because of the small amount of liquid, the small and medium batches will not need to be thickened. Simply remove the saucepan from the heat.

7. For the large batch, whisk the water and cornstarch in a small bowl until smooth, then whisk this slurry into the soy or tamari mixture in the saucepan. Cook about 1 minute, whisking constantly, until thickened. Remove from the heat.

8. When the cauliflower florets are done, dump them into a large bowl. Pour the mixture in the saucepan over them. Toss well to coat. Serve warm.

Roasted Brussels Sprouts With Bacon

Cooking Time: 20 Minutes

Servings: 4

Ingredients:

- 4 slices thick-cut bacon, chopped (about ¼ pound)
- 1 pound Brussels sprouts, halved (or quartered if large)
- freshly ground black pepper

Directions:

1. Preheat the air fryer to 380°F.
2. Air-fry the bacon for 5 minutes, shaking the basket once or twice during the cooking time.
3. Add the Brussels sprouts to the basket and drizzle a little bacon fat from the bottom of the air fryer drawer into the basket. Toss the sprouts to coat with the bacon fat. Air-fry for an additional 15 minutes, or until the Brussels sprouts are tender to a knifepoint.
4. Season with freshly ground black pepper.

Roasted Eggplant Halves With Herbed Ricotta

Servings: 3

Cooking Time: 20 Minutes

Ingredients:

- 3 5- to 6-ounce small eggplants, stemmed
- Olive oil spray
- ¼ teaspoon Table salt
- ¼ teaspoon Ground black pepper
- ½ cup Regular or low-fat ricotta
- 1½ tablespoons Minced fresh basil leaves
- 1¼ teaspoons Minced fresh oregano leaves
- Honey

Directions:

1. Preheat the air fryer to 325°F (or 330°F, if that's the closest setting).

2. Cut the eggplants in half lengthwise. Set them cut side up on your work surface. Using the tip of a paring knife, make a series of slits about three-quarters down into the flesh of each eggplant half; work at a 45-degree angle to the (former) stem across the vegetable and make the slits about ½ inch apart. Make a second set of equidistant slits at a 90-degree angle to the first slits, thus creating a crosshatch pattern in the vegetable.

3. Generously coat the cut sides of the eggplants with olive oil spray. Sprinkle the salt and pepper over the cut surfaces.

4. Set the eggplant halves cut side up in the basket with as much air space between them as possible. Air-fry undisturbed for 20 minutes, or until soft and golden.

5. Use kitchen tongs to gently transfer the eggplant halves to serving plates or a platter. Cool for 5 minutes.

6. Whisk the ricotta, basil, and oregano in a small bowl until well combined. Top the eggplant halves with this mixture. Drizzle the halves with honey to taste before serving warm.

Hush Puppies

| Servings: 8 | Cooking Time: 11 Minutes |

Ingredients:

- ½ cup Whole or low-fat milk (not fat-free)
- 1½ tablespoons Butter
- ½ cup plus 1 tablespoon, plus more All-purpose flour
- ½ cup plus 1 tablespoon Yellow cornmeal
- 2 teaspoons Granulated white sugar
- 2 teaspoons Baking powder
- ¾ teaspoon Baking soda
- ¾ teaspoon Table salt
- ¼ teaspoon Onion powder
- 3 tablespoons (or 1 medium egg, well beaten) Pasteurized egg substitute, such as Egg Beaters
- Vegetable oil spray

Directions:

1. Heat the milk and butter in a small saucepan set over medium heat just until the butter melts and the milk is steamy. Do not simmer or boil.

2. Meanwhile, whisk the flour, cornmeal, sugar, baking powder, baking soda, salt, and onion powder in a large bowl until the mixture is a uniform color.

3. Stir the hot milk mixture into the flour mixture to form a dough. Set aside to cool for 5 minutes.

4. Mix the egg substitute or egg into the dough to make a thick, smooth batter. Cover and refrigerate for at least 1 hour or up to 4 hours.

5. Preheat the air fryer to 350°F .

6. Lightly flour your clean, dry hands. Roll 2 tablespoons of the batter into a ball between your floured palms. Set aside, flour your hands again if necessary, and continue making more balls with the remaining batter.

7. Coat the balls all over with the vegetable oil spray. Line the machine's basket (or basket attachment) with a piece of parchment paper. Set the balls on the parchment paper with as much air space between them as possible. Air-fry for 9 minutes, or until lightly browned and set.

8. Use kitchen tongs to gently transfer the hush puppies to a wire rack. Cool for at least 5 minutes before serving. Or cool to room temperature, about 45 minutes, and store in a sealed container at room temperature for up to 2 days. To crisp the hush puppies again, put them in a 350°F air fryer for 2 minutes. (There's no need for parchment paper in the machine during reheating.)

Buttery Rolls

Servings: 6   Cooking Time: 14 Minutes

Ingredients:

- 6½ tablespoons Room-temperature whole or low-fat milk
- 3 tablespoons plus 1 teaspoon Butter, melted and cooled
- 3 tablespoons plus 1 teaspoon (or 1 medium egg, well beaten) Pasteurized egg substitute, such as Egg Beaters
- 1½ tablespoons Granulated white sugar
- 1¼ teaspoons Instant yeast
- ¼ teaspoon Table salt
- 2 cups, plus more for dusting All-purpose flour
- Vegetable oil
- Additional melted butter, for brushing

Directions:

1. Stir the milk, melted butter, pasteurized egg substitute (or whole egg), sugar, yeast, and salt in a medium bowl to combine. Stir in the flour just until the mixture makes a soft dough.

2. Lightly flour a clean, dry work surface. Turn the dough out onto the work surface. Knead the dough for 5 minutes to develop the gluten.

3. Lightly oil the inside of a clean medium bowl. Gather the dough into a compact ball and set it in the bowl. Turn the dough over so that its surface has oil on it all over. Cover the bowl tightly with plastic wrap and set aside in a warm, draft-free place until the dough has doubled in bulk, about 1½ hours.

4. Punch down the dough, then turn it out onto a clean, dry work surface. Divide it into 5 even balls for a small batch, 6 balls for a medium batch, or 8 balls for a large one.

5. For a small batch, lightly oil the inside of a 6-inch round cake pan and set the balls around its perimeter, separating them as much as possible.

6. For a medium batch, lightly oil the inside of a 7-inch round cake pan and set the balls in it with one ball at its center, separating them as much as possible.

7. For a large batch, lightly oil the inside of an 8-inch round cake pan and set the balls in it with one at the center, separating them as much as possible.

8. Cover with plastic wrap and set aside to rise for 30 minutes.

9. Preheat the air fryer to 350°F .

10. Uncover the pan and brush the rolls with a little melted butter, perhaps ½ teaspoon per roll. When the machine is at temperature, set the cake pan in the basket. Air-fry undisturbed for 14 minutes, or until the rolls have risen and browned.

11. Using kitchen tongs and a nonstick-safe spatula, two hot pads, or silicone baking mitts, transfer the cake pan from the basket to a wire rack. Cool the rolls in the pan for a minute or two. Turn the rolls out onto a wire rack, set them top side up again, and cool for at least another couple of minutes before serving warm.

Homemade Potato Puffs

Servings: 4

Cooking Time: 15 Minutes

Ingredients:

- 1¾ cups Water
- 4 tablespoons (¼ cup/½ stick) Butter
- 2 cups plus 2 tablespoons Instant mashed potato flakes
- 1½ teaspoons Table salt
- ¾ teaspoon Ground black pepper
- ¼ teaspoon Mild paprika
- ¼ teaspoon Dried thyme
- 1¼ cups Seasoned Italian-style dried bread crumbs (gluten-free, if a concern)
- Olive oil spray

Directions:

1. Heat the water with the butter in a medium saucepan set over medium-low heat just until the butter melts. Do not bring to a boil.

2. Remove the saucepan from the heat and stir in the potato flakes, salt, pepper, paprika, and thyme until smooth. Set aside to cool for 5 minutes.

3. Preheat the air fryer to 400°F. Spread the bread crumbs on a dinner plate.

4. Scrape up 2 tablespoons of the potato flake mixture and form it into a small, oblong puff, like a little cylinder about 1½ inches long. Gently roll the puff in the bread crumbs until coated on all sides. Set it aside and continue making more, about 12 for the small batch, 18 for the medium batch, or 24 for the large.

5. Coat the potato cylinders with olive oil spray on all sides, then arrange them in the basket in one layer with some air space between them. Air-fry undisturbed for 15 minutes, or until crisp and brown.

6. Gently dump the contents of the basket onto a wire rack. Cool for 5 minutes before serving.

Cheesy Potato Pot

Servings: 4

Cooking Time: 13 Minutes

Ingredients:

- 3 cups cubed red potatoes (unpeeled, cut into ½-inch cubes)
- ½ teaspoon garlic powder
- salt and pepper
- 1 tablespoon oil
- chopped chives for garnish (optional)
- Sauce
- 2 tablespoons milk
- 1 tablespoon butter
- 2 ounces sharp Cheddar cheese, grated
- 1 tablespoon sour cream

Directions:

1. Place potato cubes in large bowl and sprinkle with garlic, salt, and pepper. Add oil and stir to coat well.

2. Cook at 390°F for 13 minutes or until potatoes are tender. Stir every 4 or 5minutes during cooking time.

3. While potatoes are cooking, combine milk and butter in a small saucepan. Warm over medium-low heat to melt butter. Add cheese and stir until it melts. The melted cheese will remain separated from the milk mixture. Remove from heat until potatoes are done.

4. When ready to serve, add sour cream to cheese mixture and stir over medium-low heat just until warmed. Place cooked potatoes in serving bowl. Pour sauce over potatoes and stir to combine.

5. Garnish with chives if desired.

Hasselback Garlic-and-butter Potatoes

Servings: 3

Cooking Time: 48 Minutes

Ingredients:

- ➢ 3 8-ounce russet potatoes
- ➢ 6 Brown button or Baby Bella mushrooms, very thinly sliced
- ➢ Olive oil spray
- ➢ 3 tablespoons Butter, melted and cooled
- ➢ 1 tablespoon Minced garlic
- ➢ ¾ teaspoon Table salt
- ➢ 3 tablespoons (about ½ ounce) Finely grated Parmesan cheese

Directions:

1. Preheat the air fryer to 350°F .

2. Cut slits down the length of each potato, about three-quarters down into the potato and spaced about ¼ inch apart. Wedge a thin mushroom slice in each slit. Generously coat the potatoes on all sides with olive oil spray.

3. When the machine is at temperature, set the potatoes mushroom side up in the basket with as much air space between them as possible. Air-fry undisturbed for 45 minutes, or tender when pricked with a fork.

4. Increase the machine's temperature to 400°F. Use kitchen tongs, and perhaps a flatware fork for balance, to gently transfer the potatoes to a cutting board. Brush each evenly with butter, then sprinkle the minced garlic and salt over them. Sprinkle the cheese evenly over the potatoes.

5. Use those same tongs to gently transfer the potatoes cheese side up to the basket in one layer with some space for air flow between them. Air-fry undisturbed for 3 minutes, or until the cheese has melted and begun to brown.

6. Use those same tongs to gently transfer the potatoes back to the wire rack. Cool for 5 minutes before serving.

Brussels Sprout And Ham Salad

Servings: 3

Cooking Time: 12 Minutes

Ingredients:

- ➤ 1 pound 2-inch-in-length Brussels sprouts, quartered through the stem
- ➤ 6 ounces Smoked ham steak, any rind removed, diced (gluten-free, if a concern)
- ➤ ¼ teaspoon Caraway seeds
- ➤ Vegetable oil spray
- ➤ ¼ cup Brine from a jar of pickles (gluten-free, if a concern)
- ➤ ¾ teaspoon Ground black pepper

Directions:

1. Preheat the air fryer to 375°F .

2. Toss the Brussels sprout quarters, ham, and caraway seeds in a bowl until well combined. Generously coat the top of the mixture with vegetable oil spray, toss again, spray again, and repeat a couple of times until the vegetables and ham are glistening.

3. When the machine is at temperature, scrape the contents of the bowl into the basket, spreading it into as close to one layer as you can. Air-fry for 12 minutes, tossing and rearranging the pieces at least twice so that any covered or touching parts are eventually exposed to the air currents, until the Brussels sprouts are tender and a little brown at the edges.

4. Dump the contents of the basket into a serving bowl. Scrape any caraway seeds from the bottom of the basket or the tray under the basket attachment into the bowl as well. Add the pickle brine and pepper. Toss well to coat. Serve warm.

Roasted Heirloom Carrots With Orange And Thyme

Servings: 2

Cooking Time: 12 Minutes

Ingredients:

- 10 to 12 heirloom or rainbow carrots (about 1 pound), scrubbed but not peeled
- 1 teaspoon olive oil
- salt and freshly ground black pepper
- 1 tablespoon butter
- 1 teaspoon fresh orange zest
- 1 teaspoon chopped fresh thyme

Directions:

1. Preheat the air fryer to 400°F.

2. Scrub the carrots and halve them lengthwise. Toss them in the olive oil, season with salt and freshly ground black pepper and transfer to the air fryer.

3. Air-fry at 400°F for 12 minutes, shaking the basket every once in a while to rotate the carrots as they cook.

4. As soon as the carrots have finished cooking, add the butter, orange zest and thyme and toss all the ingredients together in the air fryer basket to melt the butter and coat evenly. Serve warm.

DESSERTS AND SWEETS

Maple Cinnamon Cheesecake

Servings: 4

Cooking Time: 12 Minutes

Ingredients:

- 6 sheets of cinnamon graham crackers
- 2 tablespoons butter
- 8 ounces Neufchâtel cream cheese
- 3 tablespoons pure maple syrup
- 1 large egg
- ½ teaspoon ground cinnamon
- ¼ teaspoon salt

Directions:

1. Preheat the air fryer to 350°F.

2. Place the graham crackers in a food processor and process until crushed into a flour. Mix with the butter and press into a mini air-fryer-safe pan lined at the bottom with parchment paper. Place in the air fryer and cook for 4 minutes.

3. In a large bowl, place the cream cheese and maple syrup. Use a hand mixer or stand mixer and beat together until smooth. Add in the egg, cinnamon, and salt and mix on medium speed until combined.

4. Remove the graham cracker crust from the air fryer and pour the batter into the pan.

5. Place the pan back in the air fryer, adjusting the temperature to 315°F. Cook for 18 minutes. Carefully remove when cooking completes. The top should be lightly browned and firm.

6. Keep the cheesecake in the pan and place in the refrigerator for 3 or more hours to firm up before serving.

White Chocolate Cranberry Blondies

Servings: 6

Cooking Time: 18 Minutes

Ingredients:

- ⅓ cup butter
- ½ cup sugar
- 1 teaspoon vanilla extract
- 1 large egg
- 1 cup all-purpose flour
- ½ teaspoon baking powder
- ⅛ teaspoon salt
- ¼ cup dried cranberries
- ¼ cup white chocolate chips

Directions:

1. Preheat the air fryer to 320°F.
2. In a large bowl, cream the butter with the sugar and vanilla extract. Whisk in the egg and set aside.
3. In a separate bowl, mix the flour with the baking powder and salt. Then gently mix the dry ingredients into the wet. Fold in the cranberries and chocolate chips.
4. Liberally spray an oven-safe 7-inch springform pan with olive oil and pour the batter into the pan.
5. Cook for 17 minutes or until a toothpick inserted in the center comes out clean.
6. Remove and let cool 5 minutes before serving.

S'mores Pockets

Servings: 6

Cooking Time: 5 Minutes

Ingredients:

- ➢ 12 sheets phyllo dough, thawed
- ➢ 1½ cups butter, melted
- ➢ ¾ cup graham cracker crumbs
- ➢ 1 (7-ounce) Giant Hershey's® milk chocolate bar
- ➢ 12 marshmallows, cut in half

Directions:

1. Place one sheet of the phyllo on a large cutting board. Keep the rest of the phyllo sheets covered with a slightly damp, clean kitchen towel. Brush the phyllo sheet generously with some melted butter. Place a second phyllo sheet on top of the first and brush it with more butter. Repeat with one more phyllo sheet until you have a stack of 3 phyllo sheets with butter brushed between the layers. Cover the phyllo sheets with one quarter of the graham cracker crumbs leaving a 1-inch border on one of the short ends of the rectangle. Cut the phyllo sheets lengthwise into 3 strips.

2. Take 2 of the strips and crisscross them to form a cross with the empty borders at the top and to the left. Place 2 of the chocolate rectangles in the center of the cross. Place 4 of the marshmallow halves on top of the chocolate. Now fold the pocket together by folding the bottom phyllo strip up over the chocolate and marshmallows. Then fold the right side over, then the top strip down and finally the left side over. Brush all the edges generously with melted butter to seal shut. Repeat with the next three sheets of phyllo, until all the sheets have been used. You will be able to make 2 pockets with every second batch because you will have an extra graham cracker crumb strip from the previous set of sheets.

3. Preheat the air fryer to 350°F.

4. Transfer 3 pockets at a time to the air fryer basket. Air-fry at 350°F for 4 to 5 minutes, until the phyllo dough is light brown in color. Flip the pockets over halfway through the cooking process. Repeat with the remaining 3 pockets.

5. Serve warm.

Giant Oatmeal–peanut Butter Cookie

Servings: 4

Cooking Time: 18 Minutes

Ingredients:

- ➤ 1 cup Rolled oats (not quick-cooking or steel-cut oats)
- ➤ ½ cup All-purpose flour
- ➤ ½ teaspoon Ground cinnamon
- ➤ ½ teaspoon Baking soda
- ➤ ⅓ cup Packed light brown sugar
- ➤ ¼ cup Solid vegetable shortening
- ➤ 2 tablespoons Natural-style creamy peanut butter
- ➤ 3 tablespoons Granulated white sugar
- ➤ 2 tablespoons (or 1 small egg, well beaten) Pasteurized egg substitute, such as Egg Beaters
- ➤ ⅓ cup Roasted, salted peanuts, chopped
- ➤ Baking spray

Directions:

1. Preheat the air fryer to 350°F .

2. Stir the oats, flour, cinnamon, and baking soda in a bowl until well combined.

3. Using an electric hand mixer at medium speed, beat the brown sugar, shortening, peanut butter, granulated white sugar, and egg substitute or egg (as applicable) until smooth and creamy, about 3 minutes, scraping down the inside of the bowl occasionally.

4. Scrape down and remove the beaters. Fold in the flour mixture and peanuts with a rubber spatula just until all the flour is moistened and the peanut bits are evenly distributed in the dough.

5. For a small air fryer, coat the inside of a 6-inch round cake pan with baking spray. For a medium air fryer, coat the inside of a 7-inch round cake pan with baking spray. And for a large air fryer, coat the inside of an 8-inch round cake pan with baking spray. Scrape and gently press the dough into the prepared pan, spreading it into an even layer to the perimeter.

6. Set the pan in the basket and air-fry undisturbed for 18 minutes, or until well browned.

7. Transfer the pan to a wire rack and cool for 15 minutes. Loosen the cookie from the perimeter with a spatula, then invert the pan onto a cutting board and let the cookie come free. Remove the pan and reinvert the cookie onto the wire rack. Cool for 5 minutes more before slicing into wedges to serve.

Peanut Butter Cup Doughnut Holes

Servings: 24   Cooking Time: 4 Minutes

Ingredients:

- 1½ cups bread flour
- 1 teaspoon active dry yeast
- 1 tablespoon sugar
- ¼ teaspoon salt
- ½ cup warm milk
- ½ teaspoon vanilla extract
- 2 egg yolks
- 2 tablespoons melted butter
- 24 miniature peanut butter cups, plus a few more for garnish
- vegetable oil, in a spray bottle
- Doughnut Topping
- 1 cup chocolate chips
- 2 tablespoons milk

Directions:

1. Combine the flour, yeast, sugar and salt in a bowl. Add the milk, vanilla, egg yolks and butter. Mix well until the dough starts to come together. Transfer the dough to a floured surface and knead by hand for 2 minutes. Shape the dough into a ball and transfer it to a large oiled bowl. Cover the bowl with a towel and let the dough rise in a warm place for 1 to 1½ hours, until the dough has doubled in size.

2. When the dough has risen, punch it down and roll it into a 24-inch long log. Cut the dough into 24 pieces. Push a peanut butter cup into the center of each piece of dough, pinch the dough shut and roll it into a ball. Place the dough balls on a cookie sheet and let them rise in a warm place for 30 minutes.

3. Preheat the air fryer to 400°F.

4. Spray or brush the dough balls lightly with vegetable oil. Air-fry eight at a time, at 400°F for 4 minutes, turning them over halfway through the cooking process.

5. While the doughnuts are air frying, prepare the topping. Place the chocolate chips and milk in a microwave safe bowl. Microwave on high for 1 minute. Stir and microwave for an additional 30 seconds if necessary to get all the chips to melt. Stir until the chips are melted and smooth.

6. Dip the top half of the doughnut holes into the melted chocolate. Place them on a rack to set up for just a few minutes and watch them disappear.

Puff Pastry Apples

Servings: 4   Cooking Time: 10 Minutes

Ingredients:

- 3 Rome or Gala apples, peeled
- 2 tablespoons sugar
- 1 teaspoon all-purpose flour
- 1 teaspoon ground cinnamon
- ⅛ teaspoon ground ginger
- pinch ground nutmeg
- 1 sheet puff pastry
- 1 tablespoon butter, cut into 4 pieces
- 1 egg, beaten
- vegetable oil
- vanilla ice cream (optional)
- caramel sauce (optional)

Directions:

1. Remove the core from the apple by cutting the four sides off the apple around the core. Slice the pieces of apple into thin half-moons, about ¼-inch thick. Combine the sugar, flour, cinnamon, ginger, and nutmeg in a large bowl. Add the apples to the bowl and gently toss until the apples are evenly coated with the spice mixture. Set aside.

2. Cut the puff pastry sheet into a 12-inch by 12-inch square. Then quarter the sheet into four 6-inch squares. Save any remaining pastry for decorating the apples at the end.

3. Divide the spiced apples between the four puff pastry squares, stacking the apples in the center of each square and placing them flat on top of each other in a circle. Top the apples with a piece of the butter.

4. Brush the four edges of the pastry with the egg wash. Bring the four corners of the pastry together, wrapping them around the apple slices and pinching them together at the top in the style of a "beggars purse" appetizer. Fold the ends of the pastry corners down onto the apple making them look like leaves. Brush the entire apple with the egg wash.

5. Using the leftover dough, make leaves to decorate the apples. Cut out 8 leaf shapes, about 1½-inches long, "drawing" the leaf veins on the pastry leaves with a paring knife. Place 2 leaves on the top of each apple, tucking the ends of the leaves under the pastry in the center of the apples. Brush the top of the leaves with additional egg wash. Sprinkle the entire apple with some granulated sugar.

6. Preheat the air fryer to 350°F.

7. Spray or brush the inside of the air fryer basket with oil. Place the apples in the basket and air-fry for 6 minutes. Carefully turn the apples over – it's easiest to remove one apple, then flip the others over and finally return the last apple to the air fryer. Air-fry for an additional 4 minutes.

8. Serve the puff pastry apples warm with vanilla ice cream and drizzle with some caramel sauce.

Coconut-custard Pie

Servings: 4

Cooking Time: 20 Minutes

Ingredients:

- 1 cup milk
- ¼ cup plus 2 tablespoons sugar
- ¼ cup biscuit baking mix
- 1 teaspoon vanilla
- 2 eggs
- 2 tablespoons melted butter
- cooking spray
- ½ cup shredded, sweetened coconut

Directions:

1. Place all ingredients except coconut in a medium bowl.
2. Using a hand mixer, beat on high speed for 3minutes.
3. Let sit for 5minutes.
4. Preheat air fryer to 330°F.
5. Spray a 6-inch round or 6 x 6-inch square baking pan with cooking spray and place pan in air fryer basket.
6. Pour filling into pan and sprinkle coconut over top.
7. Cook pie at 330°F for 20 minutes or until center sets.

Oreo-coated Peanut Butter Cups

Servings:8

Cooking Time: 4 Minutes

Ingredients:

- 8 Standard ¾-ounce peanut butter cups, frozen
- ⅓ cup All-purpose flour
- 2 Large egg white(s), beaten until foamy
- 16 Oreos or other creme-filled chocolate sandwich cookies, ground to crumbs in a food processor
- Vegetable oil spray

Directions:

1. Set up and fill three shallow soup plates or small pie plates on your counter: one for the flour, one for the beaten egg white(s), and one for the cookie crumbs.

2. Dip a frozen peanut butter cup in the flour, turning it to coat all sides. Shake off any excess, then set it in the beaten egg white(s). Turn it to coat all sides, then let any excess egg white slip back into the rest. Set the candy bar in the cookie crumbs. Turn to coat on all parts, even the sides. Dip the peanut butter cup back in the egg white(s) as before, then into the cookie crumbs as before, making sure you have a solid, even coating all around the cup. Set aside while you dip and coat the remaining cups.

3. When all the peanut butter cups are dipped and coated, lightly coat them on all sides with the vegetable oil spray. Set them on a plate and freeze while the air fryer heats.

4. Preheat the air fryer to 400°F.

5. Set the dipped cups wider side up in the basket with as much air space between them as possible. Air-fry undisturbed for 4 minutes, or until they feel soft but the coating is set.

6. Turn off the machine and remove the basket from it. Set aside the basket with the fried cups for 10 minutes. Use a nonstick-safe spatula to transfer the fried cups to a wire rack. Cool for at least another 5 minutes before serving.

Baked Apple Crisp

Servings: 4

Cooking Time: 23 Minutes

Ingredients:

- 2 large Granny Smith apples, peeled, cored, and chopped
- ¼ cup granulated sugar
- ¼ cup plus 2 teaspoons flour, divided
- 2 teaspoons milk
- ¼ teaspoon cinnamon
- ¼ cup oats
- ¼ cup brown sugar
- 2 tablespoons unsalted butter
- ⅛ teaspoon baking powder
- ⅛ teaspoon salt

Directions:

1. Preheat the air fryer to 350°F.

2. In a medium bowl, mix the apples, the granulated sugar, 2 teaspoons of the flour, the milk, and the cinnamon.

3. Spray 4 oven-safe ramekins with cooking spray. Divide the filling among the four ramekins.

4. In a small bowl, mix the oats, the brown sugar, the remaining ¼ cup of flour, the butter, the baking powder, and the salt. Use your fingers or a pastry blender to crumble the butter into pea-size pieces. Divide the topping over the top of the apple filling. Cover the apple crisps with foil.

5. Place the covered apple crisps in the air fryer basket and cook for 20 minutes. Uncover and continue cooking for 3 minutes or until the surface is golden and crunchy.

Cinnamon Sugar Banana Rolls

Servings: 6

Cooking Time: 8 Minutes

Ingredients:

- ¼ cup Granulated white sugar
- 2 teaspoons Ground cinnamon
- 2 tablespoons Peach or apricot jam or orange marmalade
- 6 Spring roll wrappers, thawed if necessary
- 2 Ripe banana(s), peeled and cut into 3-inch-long sections
- 1 Large egg, well beaten
- Vegetable oil spray

Directions:

1. Preheat the air fryer to 400°F.

2. Stir the sugar and cinnamon in a small bowl until well combined. Stir the jam or marmalade with a fork to loosen it up.

3. Set a spring roll wrapper on a clean, dry work surface. Roll a banana section in the sugar mixture until evenly and well coated. Set the coated banana along one edge of the wrapper. Top it with about 1 teaspoon of the jam or marmalade. Fold the sides of the wrapper perpendicular to the banana up and over the banana, partially covering it. Brush beaten egg over the side of the wrapper farthest from the banana. Starting with the banana, roll the wrapper closed, ending at the part with the beaten egg. Press gently to seal. Set the roll aside seam side down and continue filling and rolling the remaining wrappers in the same way.

4. Lightly coat the wrappers with vegetable oil spray. Set them seam side down in the basket with as much air space between them as possible. Air-fry undisturbed for 8 minutes, or until crisp and golden brown.

5. Use kitchen tongs to gently transfer the rolls to a wire rack. Cool for at least 5 minutes or up to 30 minutes before serving.

Dark Chocolate Peanut Butter S'mores

Servings: 4

Cooking Time: 6 Minutes

Ingredients:

- 4 graham cracker sheets
- 4 marshmallows
- 4 teaspoons chunky peanut butter
- 4 ounces dark chocolate
- ½ teaspoon ground cinnamon

Directions:

1. Preheat the air fryer to 390°F. Break the graham crackers in half so you have 8 pieces.

2. Place 4 pieces of graham cracker on the bottom of the air fryer. Top each with one of the marshmallows and bake for 6 or 7 minutes, or until the marshmallows have a golden brown center.

3. While cooking, slather each of the remaining graham crackers with 1 teaspoon peanut butter.

4. When baking completes, carefully remove each of the graham crackers, add 1 ounce of dark chocolate on top of the marshmallow, and lightly sprinkle with cinnamon. Top with the remaining peanut butter graham cracker to make the sandwich. Serve immediately.

Fried Snickers Bars

Servings:8

Cooking Time: 4 Minutes

Ingredients:

- ⅓ cup All-purpose flour
- 1 Large egg white(s), beaten until foamy
- 1½ cups (6 ounces) Vanilla wafer cookie crumbs
- 8 Fun-size (0.6-ounce/17-gram) Snickers bars, frozen
- Vegetable oil spray

Directions:

1. Preheat the air fryer to 400°F.

2. Set up and fill three shallow soup plates or small pie plates on your counter: one for the flour, one for the beaten egg white(s), and one for the cookie crumbs.

3. Unwrap the frozen candy bars. Dip one in the flour, turning it to coat on all sides. Gently shake off any excess, then set it in the beaten egg white(s). Turn it to coat all sides, even the ends, then let any excess egg white slip back into the rest. Set the candy bar in the cookie crumbs. Turn to coat on all sides, even the ends. Dip the candy bar back in the egg white(s) a second time, then into the cookie crumbs a second time, making sure you have an even coating all around. Coat the covered candy bar all over with vegetable oil spray. Set aside so you can dip and coat the remaining candy bars.

4. Set the coated candy bars in the basket with as much air space between them as possible. Air-fry undisturbed for 4 minutes, or until golden brown.

5. Remove the basket from the machine and let the candy bars cool in the basket for 10 minutes. Use a nonstick-safe spatula to transfer them to a wire rack and cool for 5 minutes more before chowing down.

BREAD AND BREAKFAST

Baked Eggs

Servings: 4

Cooking Time: 6 Minutes

Ingredients:

- 4 large eggs
- ⅛ teaspoon black pepper
- ⅛ teaspoon salt

Directions:

1. Preheat the air fryer to 330°F. Place 4 silicone muffin liners into the air fryer basket.
2. Crack 1 egg at a time into each silicone muffin liner. Sprinkle with black pepper and salt.
3. Bake for 6 minutes. Remove and let cool 2 minutes prior to serving.

Apple Fritters

Servings: 6

Cooking Time: 12 Minutes

Ingredients:

- 1 cup all-purpose flour
- 1½ teaspoons baking powder
- ¼ teaspoon salt
- 2 tablespoon brown sugar
- 1 teaspoon vanilla extract
- ¾ cup plain Greek yogurt
- 1 tablespoon cinnamon
- 1 large Granny Smith apple, cored, peeled, and finely chopped
- ¼ cup chopped walnuts
- ½ cup powdered sugar
- 1 tablespoon milk

Directions:

1. Preheat the air fryer to 320°F.

2. In a medium bowl, combine the flour, baking powder, and salt.

3. In a large bowl, add the brown sugar, vanilla, yogurt, cinnamon, apples, and walnuts. Mix the dry ingredients into the wet, using your hands to combine, until all the ingredients are mixed together. Knead the mixture in the bowl about 4 times.

4. Lightly spray the air fryer basket with olive oil spray.

5. Divide the batter into 6 equally sized balls; then lightly flatten them and place inside the basket. Repeat until all the fritters are formed.

6. Place the basket in the air fryer and cook for 6 minutes, flip, and then cook another 6 minutes.

7. While the fritters are cooking, in a small bowl, mix the powdered sugar with the milk. Set aside.

8. When the cooking completes, remove the air fryer basket and allow the fritters to cool on a wire rack. Drizzle with the homemade glaze and serve.

Egg Muffins

Servings: 4

Cooking Time: 11 Minutes

Ingredients:

- ➢ 4 eggs
- ➢ salt and pepper
- ➢ olive oil
- ➢ 4 English muffins, split
- ➢ 1 cup shredded Colby Jack cheese
- ➢ 4 slices ham or Canadian bacon

Directions:

1. Preheat air fryer to 390°F.

2. Beat together eggs and add salt and pepper to taste. Spray air fryer baking pan lightly with oil and add eggs. Cook for 2minutes, stir, and continue cooking for 4minutes, stirring every minute, until eggs are scrambled to your preference. Remove pan from air fryer.

3. Place bottom halves of English muffins in air fryer basket. Take half of the shredded cheese and divide it among the muffins. Top each with a slice of ham and one-quarter of the eggs. Sprinkle remaining cheese on top of the eggs. Use a fork to press the cheese into the egg a little so it doesn't slip off before it melts.

4. Cook at 360°F for 1 minute. Add English muffin tops and cook for 4minutes to heat through and toast the muffins.

Quiche Cups

Servings: 10

Cooking Time: 16 Minutes

Ingredients:

- ¼ pound all-natural ground pork sausage
- 3 eggs
- ¾ cup milk
- 20 foil muffin cups
- cooking spray
- 4 ounces sharp Cheddar cheese, grated

Directions:

1. Divide sausage into 3 portions and shape each into a thin patty.
2. Place patties in air fryer basket and cook 390°F for 6minutes.
3. While sausage is cooking, prepare the egg mixture. A large measuring cup or bowl with a pouring lip works best. Combine the eggs and milk and whisk until well blended. Set aside.
4. When sausage has cooked fully, remove patties from basket, drain well, and use a fork to crumble the meat into small pieces.
5. Double the foil cups into 10 sets. Remove paper liners from the top muffin cups and spray the foil cups lightly with cooking spray.
6. Divide crumbled sausage among the 10 muffin cup sets.
7. Top each with grated cheese, divided evenly among the cups.
8. Place 5 cups in air fryer basket.
9. Pour egg mixture into each cup, filling until each cup is at least ⅔ full.
10. Cook for 8 minutes and test for doneness. A knife inserted into the center shouldn't have any raw egg on it when removed.
11. If needed, cook 2 more minutes, until egg completely sets.
12. Repeat steps 8 through 11 for the remaining quiches.

Southwest Cornbread

Servings: 6

Cooking Time: 18 Minutes

Ingredients:

- cooking spray
- ½ cup yellow cornmeal
- ½ cup flour
- 2 teaspoons baking powder
- ½ teaspoon salt
- ½ cup frozen corn kernels, thawed and drained
- ¼ cup finely chopped onion
- 1 or 2 small jalapeño peppers, seeded and chopped
- 1 egg
- ½ cup milk
- 2 tablespoons melted butter
- 2 ounces sharp Cheddar cheese, grated

Directions:

1. Preheat air fryer to 360°F.
2. Spray air fryer baking pan with nonstick cooking spray.
3. In a medium bowl, stir together the cornmeal, flour, baking powder, and salt.
4. Stir in the corn, onion, and peppers.
5. In a small bowl, beat together the egg, milk, and butter. Stir into dry ingredients until well combined.
6. Spoon half the batter into prepared baking pan, spreading to edges. Top with grated cheese. Spoon remaining batter on top of cheese and gently spread to edges of pan so it completely covers the cheese.
7. Cook at 360°F for 18 minutes, until cornbread is done and top is crispy brown.

Blueberry Muffins

Servings: 8

Cooking Time: 14 Minutes

Ingredients:

- 1⅓ cups flour
- ½ cup sugar
- 2 teaspoons baking powder
- ¼ teaspoon salt
- ⅓ cup canola oil
- 1 egg
- ½ cup milk
- ⅔ cup blueberries, fresh or frozen and thawed
- 8 foil muffin cups including paper liners

Directions:

1. Preheat air fryer to 330°F.
2. In a medium bowl, stir together flour, sugar, baking powder, and salt.
3. In a separate bowl, combine oil, egg, and milk and mix well.
4. Add egg mixture to dry ingredients and stir just until moistened.
5. Gently stir in blueberries.
6. Spoon batter evenly into muffin cups.
7. Place 4 muffin cups in air fryer basket and bake at 330°F for 14 minutes or until tops spring back when touched lightly.
8. Repeat previous step to cook remaining muffins.

Spinach And Artichoke White Pizza

Servings: 2

Cooking Time: 18 Minutes

Ingredients:

- ➢ olive oil
- ➢ 3 cups fresh spinach
- ➢ 2 cloves garlic, minced, divided
- ➢ 1 (6- to 8-ounce) pizza dough ball*
- ➢ ½ cup grated mozzarella cheese
- ➢ ¼ cup grated Fontina cheese
- ➢ ¼ cup artichoke hearts, coarsely chopped
- ➢ 2 tablespoons grated Parmesan cheese
- ➢ ¼ teaspoon dried oregano
- ➢ salt and freshly ground black pepper

Directions:

1. Heat the oil in a medium sauté pan on the stovetop. Add the spinach and half the minced garlic to the pan and sauté for a few minutes, until the spinach has wilted. Remove the sautéed spinach from the pan and set it aside.

2. Preheat the air fryer to 390°F.

3. Cut out a piece of aluminum foil the same size as the bottom of the air fryer basket. Brush the foil circle with olive oil. Shape the dough into a circle and place it on top of the foil. Dock the dough by piercing it several times with a fork. Brush the dough lightly with olive oil and transfer it into the air fryer basket with the foil on the bottom.

4. Air-fry the plain pizza dough for 6 minutes. Turn the dough over, remove the aluminum foil and brush again with olive oil. Air-fry for an additional 4 minutes.

5. Sprinkle the mozzarella and Fontina cheeses over the dough. Top with the spinach and artichoke hearts. Sprinkle the Parmesan cheese and dried oregano on top and drizzle with olive oil. Lower the temperature of the air fryer to 350°F and cook for 8 minutes, until the cheese has melted and is lightly browned. Season to taste with salt and freshly ground black pepper.

Ham And Cheddar Gritters

Servings: 6

Cooking Time: 12 Minutes

Ingredients:

- ➢ 4 cups water
- ➢ 1 cup quick-cooking grits
- ➢ ¼ teaspoon salt
- ➢ 2 tablespoons butter
- ➢ 2 cups grated Cheddar cheese, divided
- ➢ 1 cup finely diced ham
- ➢ 1 tablespoon chopped chives
- ➢ salt and freshly ground black pepper
- ➢ 1 egg, beaten
- ➢ 2 cups panko breadcrumbs
- ➢ vegetable oil

Directions:

1. Bring the water to a boil in a saucepan. Whisk in the grits and ¼ teaspoon of salt, and cook for 7 minutes until the grits are soft. Remove the pan from the heat and stir in the butter and 1 cup of the grated Cheddar cheese. Transfer the grits to a bowl and let them cool for just 10 to 15 minutes.

2. Stir the ham, chives and the rest of the cheese into the grits and season with salt and pepper to taste. Add the beaten egg and refrigerate the mixture for 30 minutes. (Try not to chill the grits much longer than 30 minutes, or the mixture will be too firm to shape into patties.)

3. While the grit mixture is chilling, make the country gravy and set it aside.

4. Place the panko breadcrumbs in a shallow dish. Measure out ¼-cup portions of the grits mixture and shape them into patties. Coat all sides of the patties with the panko breadcrumbs, patting them with your hands so the crumbs adhere to the patties. You should have about 16 patties. Spray both sides of the patties with oil.

5. Preheat the air fryer to 400°F.

6. In batches of 5 or 6, air-fry the fritters for 8 minutes. Using a flat spatula, flip the fritters over and air-fry for another 4 minutes.

7. Serve hot with country gravy.

Tuscan Toast

Servings: 4

Cooking Time: 5 Minutes

Ingredients:

- ¼ cup butter
- ½ teaspoon lemon juice
- ½ clove garlic
- ½ teaspoon dried parsley flakes
- 4 slices Italian bread, 1-inch thick

Directions:

1. Place butter, lemon juice, garlic, and parsley in a food processor. Process about 1 minute, or until garlic is pulverized and ingredients are well blended.
2. Spread garlic butter on both sides of bread slices.
3. Place bread slices upright in air fryer basket. (They can lie flat but cook better standing on end.)
4. Cook at 390°F for 5minutes or until toasty brown.

French Toast Sticks

Servings: 4

Cooking Time: 7 Minutes

Ingredients:

- 2 eggs
- ½ cup milk
- ⅛ teaspoon salt
- ½ teaspoon pure vanilla extract
- ¾ cup crushed cornflakes
- 6 slices sandwich bread, each slice cut into 4 strips
- oil for misting or cooking spray
- maple syrup or honey

Directions:

1. In a small bowl, beat together eggs, milk, salt, and vanilla.
2. Place crushed cornflakes on a plate or in a shallow dish.
3. Dip bread strips in egg mixture, shake off excess, and roll in cornflake crumbs.
4. Spray both sides of bread strips with oil.
5. Place bread strips in air fryer basket in single layer.
6. Cook at 390°F for 7minutes or until they're dark golden brown.
7. Repeat steps 5 and 6 to cook remaining French toast sticks.
8. Serve with maple syrup or honey for dipping.

Wild Blueberry Lemon Chia Bread

Servings: 6

Cooking Time: 27 Minutes

Ingredients:

- ¼ cup extra-virgin olive oil
- ⅓ cup plus 1 tablespoon cane sugar
- 1 large egg
- 3 tablespoons fresh lemon juice
- 1 tablespoon lemon zest
- ⅔ cup milk
- 1 cup all-purpose flour
- ¾ teaspoon baking powder
- ⅛ teaspoon salt
- 2 tablespoons chia seeds
- 1 cup frozen wild blueberries
- ⅓ cup powdered sugar
- 2 teaspoons milk

Directions:

1. Preheat the air fryer to 310°F.
2. In a medium bowl, mix the olive oil with the sugar. Whisk in the egg, lemon juice, lemon zest, and milk; set aside.
3. In a small bowl, combine the all-purpose flour, baking powder, and salt.
4. Slowly mix the dry ingredients into the wet ingredients. Stir in the chia seeds and wild blueberries.
5. Liberally spray a 7-inch springform pan with olive-oil spray. Pour the batter into the pan and place the pan in the air fryer. Bake for 25 to 27 minutes, or until a toothpick inserted in the center comes out clean.
6. Remove and let cool on a wire rack for 10 minutes prior to removing from the pan.
7. Meanwhile, in a small bowl, mix the powdered sugar with the milk to create the glaze.
8. Slice and serve with a drizzle of the powdered sugar glaze.

Crunchy French Toast Sticks

Servings: 2

Cooking Time: 9 Minutes

Ingredients:

- ➢ 2 eggs, beaten
- ➢ ¾ cup milk
- ➢ ½ teaspoon vanilla extract
- ➢ ½ teaspoon ground cinnamon
- ➢ 1½ cups crushed crunchy cinnamon cereal, or any cereal flakes
- ➢ 4 slices Texas Toast (or other bread that you can slice into 1-inch thick slices)
- ➢ maple syrup, for serving
- ➢ vegetable oil or melted butter

Directions:

1. Combine the eggs, milk, vanilla and cinnamon in a shallow bowl. Place the crushed cereal in a second shallow bowl.

2. Trim the crusts off the slices of bread and cut each slice into 3 sticks. Dip the sticks of bread into the egg mixture, turning them over to coat all sides. Let the bread sticks absorb the egg mixture for ten seconds or so, but don't let them get too wet. Roll the bread sticks in the cereal crumbs, pressing the cereal gently onto all sides so that it adheres to the bread.

3. Preheat the air fryer to 400°F.

4. Spray or brush the air fryer basket with oil or melted butter. Place the coated sticks in the basket. It's ok to stack a few on top of the others in the opposite direction.

5. Air-fry for 9 minutes. Turn the sticks over a couple of times during the cooking process so that the sticks crisp evenly. Serve warm with the maple syrup or some berries.

FISH AND SEAFOOD RECIPES

Fried Shrimp

Servings:3

Cooking Time: 7 Minutes

Ingredients:

- 1 Large egg white
- 2 tablespoons Water
- 1 cup Plain dried bread crumbs (gluten-free, if a concern)
- ¼ cup All-purpose flour or almond flour
- ¼ cup Yellow cornmeal
- 1 teaspoon Celery salt
- 1 teaspoon Mild paprika
- Up to ½ teaspoon Cayenne (optional)
- ¾ pound Large shrimp (20–25 per pound), peeled and deveined
- Vegetable oil spray

Directions:

1. Preheat the air fryer to 400°F.

2. Set two medium or large bowls on your counter. In the first, whisk the egg white and water until foamy. In the second, stir the bread crumbs, flour, cornmeal, celery salt, paprika, and cayenne (if using) until well combined.

3. Pour all the shrimp into the egg white mixture and stir gently until all the shrimp are coated. Use kitchen tongs to pick them up one by one and transfer them to the bread-crumb mixture. Turn each in the bread-crumb mixture to coat it evenly and thoroughly on all sides before setting it on a cutting board. When you're done coating the shrimp, coat them all on both sides with the vegetable oil spray.

4. Set the shrimp in as close to one layer in the basket as you can. Some may overlap. Air-fry for 7 minutes, gently rearranging the shrimp at the 4-minute mark to get covered surfaces exposed, until golden brown and firm but not hard.

5. Use kitchen tongs to gently transfer the shrimp to a wire rack. Cool for only a minute or two before serving.

Horseradish-crusted Salmon Fillets

Servings:3

Cooking Time: 8 Minutes

Ingredients:

- ½ cup Fresh bread crumbs (see the headnote)
- 4 tablespoons (¼ cup/½ stick) Butter, melted and cooled
- ¼ cup Jarred prepared white horseradish
- Vegetable oil spray
- 4 6-ounce skin-on salmon fillets (for more information, see here)

Directions:

1. Preheat the air fryer to 400°F.

2. Mix the bread crumbs, butter, and horseradish in a bowl until well combined.

3. Take the basket out of the machine. Generously spray the skin side of each fillet. Pick them up one by one with a nonstick-safe spatula and set them in the basket skin side down with as much air space between them as possible. Divide the bread-crumb mixture between the fillets, coating the top of each fillet with an even layer. Generously coat the bread-crumb mixture with vegetable oil spray.

4. Return the basket to the machine and air-fry undisturbed for 8 minutes, or until the topping has lightly browned and the fish is firm but not hard.

5. Use a nonstick-safe spatula to transfer the salmon fillets to serving plates. Cool for 5 minutes before serving. Because of the butter in the topping, it will stay very hot for quite a while. Take care, especially if you're serving these fillets to children.

Bacon-wrapped Scallops

Servings: 4

Cooking Time: 8 Minutes

Ingredients:

- ➢ 16 large scallops
- ➢ 8 bacon strips
- ➢ ½ teaspoon black pepper
- ➢ ¼ teaspoon smoked paprika

Directions:

1. Pat the scallops dry with a paper towel. Slice each of the bacon strips in half. Wrap 1 bacon strip around 1 scallop and secure with a toothpick. Repeat with the remaining scallops. Season the scallops with pepper and paprika.

2. Preheat the air fryer to 350°F.

3. Place the bacon-wrapped scallops in the air fryer basket and cook for 4 minutes, shake the basket, cook another 3 minutes, shake the basket, and cook another 1 to 3 to minutes. When the bacon is crispy, the scallops should be cooked through and slightly firm, but not rubbery. Serve immediately.

Shrimp Teriyaki

Servings:10

Cooking Time: 6 Minutes

Ingredients:

- ➢ 1 tablespoon Regular or low-sodium soy sauce or gluten-free tamari sauce
- ➢ 1 tablespoon Mirin or a substitute (see here)
- ➢ 1 teaspoon Ginger juice (see the headnote)
- ➢ 10 Large shrimp (20–25 per pound), peeled and deveined
- ➢ ⅔ cup Plain panko bread crumbs (gluten-free, if a concern)
- ➢ 1 Large egg
- ➢ Vegetable oil spray

Directions:

1. Whisk the soy or tamari sauce, mirin, and ginger juice in an 8- or 9-inch square baking pan until uniform. Add the shrimp and toss well to coat. Cover and refrigerate for 1 hour, tossing the shrimp in the marinade at least twice.

2. Preheat the air fryer to 400°F.

3. Thread a marinated shrimp on a 4-inch bamboo skewer by inserting the pointy tip at the small end of the shrimp, then guiding the skewer along the shrimp so that the tip comes out the thick end and the shrimp is flat along the length of the skewer. Repeat with the remaining shrimp. (You'll need eight 4-inch skewers for the small batch, 10 skewers for the medium batch, and 12 for the large.)

4. Pour the bread crumbs onto a dinner plate. Whisk the egg in the baking pan with any marinade that stayed behind. Lay the skewers in the pan, in as close to a single layer as possible. Turn repeatedly to make sure the shrimp is coated in the egg mixture.

5. One at a time, take a skewered shrimp out of the pan and set it in the bread crumbs, turning several times and pressing gently until the shrimp is evenly coated on all sides. Coat the shrimp with vegetable oil spray and set the skewer aside. Repeat with the remainder of the shrimp.

6. Set the skewered shrimp in the basket in one layer. Air-fry undisturbed for 6 minutes, or until pink and firm.

7. Transfer the skewers to a wire rack. Cool for only a minute or two before serving.

Stuffed Shrimp

Ingredients:

- 16 tail-on shrimp, peeled and deveined (last tail section intact)
- ¾ cup crushed panko breadcrumbs
- oil for misting or cooking spray
- Stuffing
- 2 6-ounce cans lump crabmeat
- 2 tablespoons chopped shallots
- 2 tablespoons chopped green onions
- 2 tablespoons chopped celery
- 2 tablespoons chopped green bell pepper
- ½ cup crushed saltine crackers
- 1 teaspoon Old Bay Seasoning
- 1 teaspoon garlic powder
- ¼ teaspoon ground thyme
- 2 teaspoons dried parsley flakes
- 2 teaspoons fresh lemon juice
- 2 teaspoons Worcestershire sauce
- 1 egg, beaten

Directions:

1. Rinse shrimp. Remove tail section (shell) from 4 shrimp, discard, and chop the meat finely.
2. To prepare the remaining 12 shrimp, cut a deep slit down the back side so that the meat lies open flat. Do not cut all the way through.
3. Preheat air fryer to 360°F.
4. Place chopped shrimp in a large bowl with all of the stuffing ingredients and stir to combine.
5. Divide stuffing into 12 portions, about 2 tablespoons each.
6. Place one stuffing portion onto the back of each shrimp and form into a ball or oblong shape. Press firmly so that stuffing sticks together and adheres to shrimp.
7. Gently roll each stuffed shrimp in panko crumbs and mist with oil or cooking spray.
8. Place 6 shrimp in air fryer basket and cook at 360°F for 10minutes. Mist with oil or spray and cook 2 minutes longer or until stuffing cooks through inside and is crispy outside.
9. Repeat step 8 to cook remaining shrimp.

Crabmeat-stuffed Flounder

Servings:3   Cooking Time: 12 Minutes

Ingredients:

- 4½ ounces Purchased backfin or claw crabmeat, picked over for bits of shell and cartilage
- 6 Saltine crackers, crushed into fine crumbs
- 2 tablespoons plus 1 teaspoon Regular or low-fat mayonnaise (not fat-free)
- ¾ teaspoon Yellow prepared mustard
- 1½ teaspoons Worcestershire sauce
- ⅛ teaspoon Celery salt
- 3 5- to 6-ounce skinless flounder fillets
- Vegetable oil spray
- Mild paprika

Directions:

1. Preheat the air fryer to 400°F.

2. Gently mix the crabmeat, crushed saltines, mayonnaise, mustard, Worcestershire sauce, and celery salt in a bowl until well combined.

3. Generously coat the flat side of a fillet with vegetable oil spray. Set the fillet sprayed side down on your work surface. Cut the fillet in half widthwise, then cut one of the halves in half lengthwise. Set a scant ⅓ cup of the crabmeat mixture on top of the undivided half of the fish fillet, mounding the mixture to make an oval that somewhat fits the shape of the fillet with at least a ¼-inch border of fillet beyond the filling all around.

4. Take the two thin divided quarters (that is, the halves of the half) and lay them lengthwise over the filling, overlapping at each end and leaving a little space in the middle where the filling peeks through. Coat the top of the stuffed flounder piece with vegetable oil spray, then sprinkle paprika over the stuffed flounder fillet. Set aside and use the remaining fillet(s) to make more stuffed flounder "packets," repeating steps 3 and

5. Use a nonstick-safe spatula to transfer the stuffed flounder fillets to the basket. Leave as much space between them as possible. Air-fry undisturbed for 12 minutes, or until lightly brown and firm (but not hard).

6. Use that same spatula, plus perhaps another one, to transfer the fillets to a serving platter or plates. Cool for a minute or two, then serve hot.

Shrimp, Chorizo And Fingerling Potatoes

Servings: 4

Cooking Time: 16 Minutes

Ingredients:

- ½ red onion, chopped into 1-inch chunks
- 8 fingerling potatoes, sliced into 1-inch slices or halved lengthwise
- 1 teaspoon olive oil
- salt and freshly ground black pepper
- 8 ounces raw chorizo sausage, sliced into 1-inch chunks
- 16 raw large shrimp, peeled, deveined and tails removed
- 1 lime
- ¼ cup chopped fresh cilantro
- chopped orange zest (optional)

Directions:

1. Preheat the air fryer to 380°F.

2. Combine the red onion and potato chunks in a bowl and toss with the olive oil, salt and freshly ground black pepper.

3. Transfer the vegetables to the air fryer basket and air-fry for 6 minutes, shaking the basket a few times during the cooking process.

4. Add the chorizo chunks and continue to air-fry for another 5 minutes.

5. Add the shrimp, season with salt and continue to air-fry, shaking the basket every once in a while, for another 5 minutes.

6. Transfer the tossed shrimp, chorizo and potato to a bowl and squeeze some lime juice over the top to taste. Toss in the fresh cilantro, orange zest and a drizzle of olive oil, and season again to taste.

7. Serve with a fresh green salad.

Shrimp "scampi"

Servings:4

Cooking Time: 5 Minutes

Ingredients:

- ➢ 1½ pounds Large shrimp (20–25 per pound), peeled and deveined
- ➢ ¼ cup Olive oil
- ➢ 2 tablespoons Minced garlic
- ➢ 1 teaspoon Dried oregano
- ➢ Up to 1 teaspoon Red pepper flakes
- ➢ ½ teaspoon Table salt
- ➢ 2 tablespoons White balsamic vinegar (see here)

Directions:

1. Preheat the air fryer to 400°F.

2. Stir the shrimp, olive oil, garlic, oregano, red pepper flakes, and salt in a large bowl until the shrimp are well coated.

3. When the machine is at temperature, transfer the shrimp to the basket. They will overlap and even sit on top of each other. Air-fry for 5 minutes, tossing and rearranging the shrimp twice to make sure the covered surfaces are exposed, until pink and firm.

4. Pour the contents of the basket into a serving bowl. Pour the vinegar over the shrimp while hot and toss to coat.

Fried Oysters

Servings:12

Cooking Time: 8 Minutes

Ingredients:

- ➢ 1½ cups All-purpose flour
- ➢ 1½ cups Yellow cornmeal
- ➢ 1½ tablespoons Cajun dried seasoning blend (for a homemade blend, see here)
- ➢ 1¼ cups, plus more if needed Amber beer, pale ale, or IPA
- ➢ 12 Large shucked oysters, any liquid drained off
- ➢ Vegetable oil spray

Directions:

1. Preheat the air fryer to 400°F.

2. Whisk ⅔ cup of the flour, ½ cup of the cornmeal, and the seasoning blend in a bowl until uniform. Set aside.

3. Whisk the remaining ⅓ cup flour and the remaining ½ cup cornmeal with the beer in a second bowl, adding more beer in dribs and drabs until the mixture is the consistency of pancake batter.

4. Using a fork, dip a shucked oyster in the beer batter, coating it thoroughly. Gently shake off any excess batter, then set the oyster in the dry mixture and turn gently to coat well and evenly. Set the coated oyster on a cutting board and continue dipping and coating the remainder of the oysters.

5. Coat the oysters with vegetable oil spray, then set them in the basket with as much air space between them as possible. Air-fry undisturbed for 8 minutes, or until lightly browned and crisp.

6. Use a nonstick-safe spatula to transfer the oysters to a wire rack. Cool for a couple of minutes before serving.

Lobster Tails With Lemon Garlic Butter

Servings: 2

Cooking Time: 5 Minutes

Ingredients:

- 4 ounces unsalted butter
- 1 tablespoon finely chopped lemon zest
- 1 clove garlic, thinly sliced
- 2 (6-ounce) lobster tails
- salt and freshly ground black pepper
- ½ cup white wine
- ½ lemon, sliced
- vegetable oil

Directions:

1. Start by making the lemon garlic butter. Combine the butter, lemon zest and garlic in a small saucepan. Melt and simmer the butter on the stovetop over the lowest possible heat while you prepare the lobster tails.

2. Prepare the lobster tails by cutting down the middle of the top of the shell. Crack the bottom shell by squeezing the sides of the lobster together so that you can access the lobster meat inside. Pull the lobster tail up out of the shell, but leave it attached at the base of the tail. Lay the lobster meat on top of the shell and season with salt and freshly ground black pepper. Pour a little of the lemon garlic butter on top of the lobster meat and transfer the lobster to the refrigerator so that the butter solidifies a little.

3. Pour the white wine into the air fryer drawer and add the lemon slices. Preheat the air fryer to 400°F for 5 minutes.

4. Transfer the lobster tails to the air fryer basket. Air-fry at 370° for 5 minutes, brushing more butter on halfway through cooking. (Add a minute or two if your lobster tail is more than 6-ounces.) Remove and serve with more butter for dipping or drizzling.

Fish Sticks For Grown-ups

Servings: 4

Cooking Time: 6 Minutes

Ingredients:

- ➤ 1 pound fish fillets
- ➤ ½ teaspoon hot sauce
- ➤ 1 tablespoon coarse brown mustard
- ➤ 1 teaspoon Worcestershire sauce
- ➤ salt
- ➤ Crumb Coating
- ➤ ¾ cup panko breadcrumbs
- ➤ ¼ cup stone-ground cornmeal
- ➤ ¼ teaspoon salt
- ➤ oil for misting or cooking spray

Directions:

1. Cut fish fillets crosswise into slices 1-inch wide.

2. Mix the hot sauce, mustard, and Worcestershire sauce together to make a paste and rub on all sides of the fish. Season to taste with salt.

3. Mix crumb coating ingredients together and spread on a sheet of wax paper.

4. Roll the fish fillets in the crumb mixture.

5. Spray all sides with olive oil or cooking spray and place in air fryer basket in a single layer.

6. Cook at 390°F for 6 minutes, until fish flakes easily.

Mahi-mahi "burrito" Fillets

Servings:3

Cooking Time: 10 Minutes

Ingredients:

- ➤ 1 Large egg white
- ➤ 1½ cups (6 ounces) Crushed corn tortilla chips (gluten-free, if a concern)
- ➤ 1 tablespoon Chile powder
- ➤ 3 5-ounce skinless mahi-mahi fillets
- ➤ 6 tablespoons Canned refried beans
- ➤ Vegetable oil spray

Directions:

1. Preheat the air fryer to 400°F.

2. Set up and fill two shallow soup plates or small pie plates on your counter: one with the egg white, beaten until foamy; and one with the crushed tortilla chips.

3. Gently rub ½ teaspoon chile powder on each side of each fillet.

4. Spread (or maybe smear) 1 tablespoon refried beans over both sides and the edges of a fillet. Dip the fillet in the egg white, turning to coat it on both sides. Let any excess egg white slip back into the rest, then set the fillet in the crushed tortilla chips. Turn several times, pressing gently to coat it evenly. Coat the fillet on all sides with the vegetable oil spray, then set it aside. Prepare the remaining fillet(s) in the same way.

5. When the machine is at temperature, set the fillets in the basket with as much air space between them as possible. Air-fry undisturbed for 10 minutes, or until crisp and browned.

6. Use a nonstick-safe spatula to transfer the fillets to a serving platter or plates. Cool for only a minute or so, then serve hot.

SANDWICHES AND BURGERS RECIPES

Chicken Saltimbocca Sandwiches

Servings: 3

Cooking Time: 11 Minutes

Ingredients:

- ➤ 3 5- to 6-ounce boneless skinless chicken breasts
- ➤ 6 Thin prosciutto slices
- ➤ 6 Provolone cheese slices
- ➤ 3 Long soft rolls, such as hero, hoagie, or Italian sub rolls (gluten-free, if a concern), split open lengthwise
- ➤ 3 tablespoons Pesto, purchased or homemade (see the headnote)

Directions:

1. Preheat the air fryer to 400°F.

2. Wrap each chicken breast with 2 prosciutto slices, spiraling the prosciutto around the breast and overlapping the slices a bit to cover the breast. The prosciutto will stick to the chicken more readily than bacon does.

3. When the machine is at temperature, set the wrapped chicken breasts in the basket and air-fry undisturbed for 10 minutes, or until the prosciutto is frizzled and the chicken is cooked through.

4. Overlap 2 cheese slices on each breast. Air-fry undisturbed for 1 minute, or until melted. Take the basket out of the machine.

5. Smear the insides of the rolls with the pesto, then use kitchen tongs to put a wrapped and cheesy chicken breast in each roll.

Thanksgiving Turkey Sandwiches

Servings: 3   Cooking Time: 10 Minutes

Ingredients:

- 1½ cups Herb-seasoned stuffing mix (not cornbread-style; gluten-free, if a concern)
- 1 Large egg white(s)
- 2 tablespoons Water
- 3 5- to 6-ounce turkey breast cutlets
- Vegetable oil spray
- 4½ tablespoons Purchased cranberry sauce, preferably whole berry
- ⅛ teaspoon Ground cinnamon
- ⅛ teaspoon Ground dried ginger
- 4½ tablespoons Regular, low-fat, or fat-free mayonnaise (gluten-free, if a concern)
- 6 tablespoons Shredded Brussels sprouts
- 3 Kaiser rolls (gluten-free, if a concern), split open

Directions:

1. Preheat the air fryer to 375°F .

2. Put the stuffing mix in a heavy zip-closed bag, seal it, lay it flat on your counter, and roll a rolling pin over the bag to crush the stuffing mix to the consistency of rough sand. (Or you can pulse the stuffing mix to the desired consistency in a food processor.)

3. Set up and fill two shallow soup plates or small pie plates on your counter: one for the egg white(s), whisked with the water until foamy; and one for the ground stuffing mix.

4. Dip a cutlet in the egg white mixture, coating both sides and letting any excess egg white slip back into the rest. Set the cutlet in the ground stuffing mix and coat it evenly on both sides, pressing gently to coat well on both sides. Lightly coat the cutlet on both sides with vegetable oil spray, set it aside, and continue dipping and coating the remaining cutlets in the same way.

5. Set the cutlets in the basket and air-fry undisturbed for 10 minutes, or until crisp and brown. Use kitchen tongs to transfer the cutlets to a wire rack to cool for a few minutes.

6. Meanwhile, stir the cranberry sauce with the cinnamon and ginger in a small bowl. Mix the shredded Brussels sprouts and mayonnaise in a second bowl until the vegetable is evenly coated.

7. Build the sandwiches by spreading about 1½ tablespoons of the cranberry mixture on the cut side of the bottom half of each roll. Set a cutlet on top, then spread about 3 tablespoons of the Brussels sprouts mixture evenly over the cutlet. Set the other half of the roll on top and serve warm.

Best-ever Roast Beef Sandwiches

Servings: 6

Cooking Time: 30-50 Minutes

Ingredients:

- ➢ 2½ teaspoons Olive oil
- ➢ 1½ teaspoons Dried oregano
- ➢ 1½ teaspoons Dried thyme
- ➢ 1½ teaspoons Onion powder
- ➢ 1½ teaspoons Table salt
- ➢ 1½ teaspoons Ground black pepper
- ➢ 3 pounds Beef eye of round
- ➢ 6 Round soft rolls, such as Kaiser rolls or hamburger buns (gluten-free, if a concern), split open lengthwise
- ➢ ¾ cup Regular, low-fat, or fat-free mayonnaise (gluten-free, if a concern)
- ➢ 6 Romaine lettuce leaves, rinsed
- ➢ 6 Round tomato slices (¼ inch thick)

Directions:

1. Preheat the air fryer to 350°F .

2. Mix the oil, oregano, thyme, onion powder, salt, and pepper in a small bowl. Spread this mixture all over the eye of round.

3. When the machine is at temperature, set the beef in the basket and air-fry for 30 to 50 minutes (the range depends on the size of the cut), turning the meat twice, until an instant-read meat thermometer inserted into the thickest piece of the meat registers 130°F for rare, 140°F for medium, or 150°F for well-done.

4. Use kitchen tongs to transfer the beef to a cutting board. Cool for 10 minutes. If serving now, carve into ⅛-inch-thick slices. Spread each roll with 2 tablespoons mayonnaise and divide the beef slices between the rolls. Top with a lettuce leaf and a tomato slice and serve. Or set the beef in a container, cover, and refrigerate for up to 3 days to make cold roast beef sandwiches anytime.

Thai-style Pork Sliders

Servings: 4

Cooking Time: 15 Minutes

Ingredients:

- ➢ 11 ounces Ground pork
- ➢ 2½ tablespoons Very thinly sliced scallions, white and green parts
- ➢ 4 teaspoons Minced peeled fresh ginger
- ➢ 2½ teaspoons Fish sauce (gluten-free, if a concern)
- ➢ 2 teaspoons Thai curry paste (see the headnote; gluten-free, if a concern)
- ➢ 2 teaspoons Light brown sugar
- ➢ ¾ teaspoon Ground black pepper
- ➢ 4 Slider buns (gluten-free, if a concern)

Directions:

1. Preheat the air fryer to 375°F .

2. Gently mix the pork, scallions, ginger, fish sauce, curry paste, brown sugar, and black pepper in a bowl until well combined. With clean, wet hands, form about ⅓ cup of the pork mixture into a slider about 2½ inches in diameter. Repeat until you use up all the meat—3 sliders for the small batch, 4 for the medium, and 6 for the large. (Keep wetting your hands to help the patties adhere.)

3. When the machine is at temperature, set the sliders in the basket in one layer. Air-fry undisturbed for 14 minutes, or until the sliders are golden brown and caramelized at their edges and an instant-read meat thermometer inserted into the center of a slider registers 160°F.

4. Use a nonstick-safe spatula, and perhaps a flatware fork for balance, to transfer the sliders to a cutting board. Set the buns cut side down in the basket in one layer (working in batches as necessary) and air-fry undisturbed for 1 minute, to toast a bit and warm up. Serve the sliders warm in the buns.

Eggplant Parmesan Subs

Servings: 2

Cooking Time: 13 Minutes

Ingredients:

- ➢ 4 Peeled eggplant slices (about ½ inch thick and 3 inches in diameter)
- ➢ Olive oil spray
- ➢ 2 tablespoons plus 2 teaspoons Jarred pizza sauce, any variety except creamy
- ➢ ¼ cup (about ⅔ ounce) Finely grated Parmesan cheese
- ➢ 2 Small, long soft rolls, such as hero, hoagie, or Italian sub rolls (gluten-free, if a concern), split open lengthwise

Directions:

1. Preheat the air fryer to 350°F .

2. When the machine is at temperature, coat both sides of the eggplant slices with olive oil spray. Set them in the basket in one layer and air-fry undisturbed for 10 minutes, until lightly browned and softened.

3. Increase the machine's temperature to 375°F (or 370°F, if that's the closest setting—unless the machine is already at 360°F, in which case leave it alone). Top each eggplant slice with 2 teaspoons pizza sauce, then 1 tablespoon cheese. Air-fry undisturbed for 2 minutes, or until the cheese has melted.

4. Use a nonstick-safe spatula, and perhaps a flatware fork for balance, to transfer the eggplant slices cheese side up to a cutting board. Set the roll(s) cut side down in the basket in one layer (working in batches as necessary) and air-fry undisturbed for 1 minute, to toast the rolls a bit and warm them up. Set 2 eggplant slices in each warm roll.

Perfect Burgers

Servings: 3

Cooking Time: 13 Minutes

Ingredients:

- ➢ 1 pound 2 ounces 90% lean ground beef
- ➢ 1½ tablespoons Worcestershire sauce (gluten-free, if a concern)
- ➢ ½ teaspoon Ground black pepper
- ➢ 3 Hamburger buns (gluten-free if a concern), split open

Directions:

1. Preheat the air fryer to 375°F .
2. Gently mix the ground beef, Worcestershire sauce, and pepper in a bowl until well combined but preserving as much of the meat's fibers as possible. Divide this mixture into two 5-inch patties for the small batch, three 5-inch patties for the medium, or four 5-inch patties for the large. Make a thumbprint indentation in the center of each patty, about halfway through the meat.
3. Set the patties in the basket in one layer with some space between them. Air-fry undisturbed for 10 minutes, or until an instant-read meat thermometer inserted into the center of a burger registers 160°F (a medium-well burger). You may need to add 2 minutes cooking time if the air fryer is at 360°F.
4. Use a nonstick-safe spatula, and perhaps a flatware fork for balance, to transfer the burgers to a cutting board. Set the buns cut side down in the basket in one layer (working in batches as necessary) and air-fry undisturbed for 1 minute, to toast a bit and warm up. Serve the burgers in the warm buns.

White Bean Veggie Burgers

Servings: 3

Cooking Time: 13 Minutes

Ingredients:

- 1⅓ cups Drained and rinsed canned white beans
- 3 tablespoons Rolled oats (not quick-cooking or steel-cut; gluten-free, if a concern)
- 3 tablespoons Chopped walnuts
- 2 teaspoons Olive oil
- 2 teaspoons Lemon juice
- 1½ teaspoons Dijon mustard (gluten-free, if a concern)
- ¾ teaspoon Dried sage leaves
- ¼ teaspoon Table salt
- Olive oil spray
- 3 Whole-wheat buns or gluten-free whole-grain buns (if a concern), split open

Directions:

1. Preheat the air fryer to 400°F.

2. Place the beans, oats, walnuts, oil, lemon juice, mustard, sage, and salt in a food processor. Cover and process to make a coarse paste that will hold its shape, about like wet sugar-cookie dough, stopping the machine to scrape down the inside of the canister at least once.

3. Scrape down and remove the blade. With clean and wet hands, form the bean paste into two 4-inch patties for the small batch, three 4-inch patties for the medium, or four 4-inch patties for the large batch. Generously coat the patties on both sides with olive oil spray.

4. Set them in the basket with some space between them and air-fry undisturbed for 12 minutes, or until lightly brown and crisp at the edges. The tops of the burgers will feel firm to the touch.

5. Use a nonstick-safe spatula, and perhaps a flatware fork for balance, to transfer the burgers to a cutting board. Set the buns cut side down in the basket in one layer (working in batches as necessary) and air-fry undisturbed for 1 minute, to toast a bit and warm up. Serve the burgers warm in the buns.

Crunchy Falafel Balls

Servings: 8

Cooking Time: 16 Minutes

Ingredients:

- 2½ cups Drained and rinsed canned chickpeas
- ¼ cup Olive oil
- 3 tablespoons All-purpose flour
- 1½ teaspoons Dried oregano
- 1½ teaspoons Dried sage leaves
- 1½ teaspoons Dried thyme
- ¾ teaspoon Table salt
- Olive oil spray

Directions:

1. Preheat the air fryer to 400°F.

2. Place the chickpeas, olive oil, flour, oregano, sage, thyme, and salt in a food processor. Cover and process into a paste, stopping the machine at least once to scrape down the inside of the canister.

3. Scrape down and remove the blade. Using clean, wet hands, form 2 tablespoons of the paste into a ball, then continue making 9 more balls for a small batch, 15 more for a medium one, and 19 more for a large batch. Generously coat the balls in olive oil spray.

4. Set the balls in the basket in one layer with a little space between them and air-fry undisturbed for 16 minutes, or until well browned and crisp.

5. Dump the contents of the basket onto a wire rack. Cool for 5 minutes before serving.

Mexican Cheeseburgers

Servings: 4

Cooking Time: 22 Minutes

Ingredients:

- ➤ 1¼ pounds ground beef
- ➤ ¼ cup finely chopped onion
- ➤ ½ cup crushed yellow corn tortilla chips
- ➤ 1 (1.25-ounce) packet taco seasoning
- ➤ ¼ cup canned diced green chilies
- ➤ 1 egg, lightly beaten
- ➤ 4 ounces pepper jack cheese, grated
- ➤ 4 (12-inch) flour tortillas
- ➤ shredded lettuce, sour cream, guacamole, salsa (for topping)

Directions:

1. Combine the ground beef, minced onion, crushed tortilla chips, taco seasoning, green chilies, and egg in a large bowl. Mix thoroughly until combined – your hands are good tools for this. Divide the meat into four equal portions and shape each portion into an oval-shaped burger.

2. Preheat the air fryer to 370°F.

3. Air-fry the burgers for 18 minutes, turning them over halfway through the cooking time. Divide the cheese between the burgers, lower fryer to 340°F and air-fry for an additional 4 minutes to melt the cheese. (This will give you a burger that is medium-well. If you prefer your cheeseburger medium-rare, shorten the cooking time to about 15 minutes and then add the cheese and proceed with the recipe.)

4. While the burgers are cooking, warm the tortillas wrapped in aluminum foil in a 350°F oven, or in a skillet with a little oil over medium-high heat for a couple of minutes. Keep the tortillas warm until the burgers are ready.

5. To assemble the burgers, spread sour cream over three quarters of the tortillas and top each with some shredded lettuce and salsa. Place the Mexican cheeseburgers on the lettuce and top with guacamole. Fold the tortillas around the burger, starting with the bottom and then folding the sides in over the top. (A little sour cream can help hold the seam of the tortilla together.) Serve immediately.

Asian Glazed Meatballs

Servings: 4

Cooking Time: 10 Minutes

Ingredients:

- 1 large shallot, finely chopped
- 2 cloves garlic, minced
- 1 tablespoon grated fresh ginger
- 2 teaspoons fresh thyme, finely chopped
- 1½ cups brown mushrooms, very finely chopped (a food processor works well here)
- 2 tablespoons soy sauce
- freshly ground black pepper
- 1 pound ground beef
- ½ pound ground pork
- 3 egg yolks
- 1 cup Thai sweet chili sauce (spring roll sauce)
- ¼ cup toasted sesame seeds
- 2 scallions, sliced

Directions:

1. Combine the shallot, garlic, ginger, thyme, mushrooms, soy sauce, freshly ground black pepper, ground beef and pork, and egg yolks in a bowl and mix the ingredients together. Gently shape the mixture into 24 balls, about the size of a golf ball.

2. Preheat the air fryer to 380°F.

3. Working in batches, air-fry the meatballs for 8 minutes, turning the meatballs over halfway through the cooking time. Drizzle some of the Thai sweet chili sauce on top of each meatball and return the basket to the air fryer, air-frying for another 2 minutes. Reserve the remaining Thai sweet chili sauce for serving.

4. As soon as the meatballs are done, sprinkle with toasted sesame seeds and transfer them to a serving platter. Scatter the scallions around and serve warm.

Chicken Club Sandwiches

Servings: 3

Cooking Time: 15 Minutes

Ingredients:

- 3 5- to 6-ounce boneless skinless chicken breasts
- 6 Thick-cut bacon strips (gluten-free, if a concern)
- 3 Long soft rolls, such as hero, hoagie, or Italian sub rolls (gluten-free, if a concern)
- 3 tablespoons Regular, low-fat, or fat-free mayonnaise (gluten-free, if a concern)
- 3 Lettuce leaves, preferably romaine or iceberg
- 6 ¼-inch-thick tomato slices

Directions:

1. Preheat the air fryer to 375°F .

2. Wrap each chicken breast with 2 strips of bacon, spiraling the bacon around the meat, slightly overlapping the strips on each revolution. Start the second strip of bacon farther down the breast but on a line with the start of the first strip so they both end at a lined-up point on the chicken breast.

3. When the machine is at temperature, set the wrapped breasts bacon-seam side down in the basket with space between them. Air-fry undisturbed for 12 minutes, until the bacon is browned, crisp, and cooked through and an instant-read meat thermometer inserted into the center of a breast registers 165°F. You may need to add 2 minutes in the air fryer if the temperature is at 360°F.

4. Use kitchen tongs to transfer the breasts to a wire rack. Split the rolls open lengthwise and set them cut side down in the basket. Air-fry for 1 minute, or until warmed through.

5. Use kitchen tongs to transfer the rolls to a cutting board. Spread 1 tablespoon mayonnaise on the cut side of one half of each roll. Top with a chicken breast, lettuce leaf, and tomato slice. Serve warm.

Chicken Spiedies

Servings: 3   Cooking Time: 12 Minutes

Ingredients:

- 1¼ pounds Boneless skinless chicken thighs, trimmed of any fat blobs and cut into 2-inch pieces
- 3 tablespoons Red wine vinegar
- 2 tablespoons Olive oil
- 2 tablespoons Minced fresh mint leaves
- 2 tablespoons Minced fresh parsley leaves
- 2 teaspoons Minced fresh dill fronds
- ¾ teaspoon Fennel seeds
- ¾ teaspoon Table salt
- Up to a ¼ teaspoon Red pepper flakes
- 3 Long soft rolls, such as hero, hoagie, or Italian sub rolls (gluten-free, if a concern), split open lengthwise
- 4½ tablespoons Regular or low-fat mayonnaise (not fat-free; gluten-free, if a concern)
- 1½ tablespoons Distilled white vinegar
- 1½ teaspoons Ground black pepper

Directions:

1. Mix the chicken, vinegar, oil, mint, parsley, dill, fennel seeds, salt, and red pepper flakes in a zip-closed plastic bag. Seal, gently massage the marinade ingredients into the meat, and refrigerate for at least 2 hours or up to 6 hours. (Longer than that and the meat can turn rubbery.)

2. Set the plastic bag out on the counter (to make the contents a little less frigid). Preheat the air fryer to 400°F.

3. When the machine is at temperature, use kitchen tongs to set the chicken thighs in the basket (discard any remaining marinade) and air-fry undisturbed for 6 minutes. Turn the thighs over and continue air-frying undisturbed for 6 minutes more, until well browned, cooked through, and even a little crunchy.

4. Dump the contents of the basket onto a wire rack and cool for 2 or 3 minutes. Divide the chicken evenly between the rolls. Whisk the mayonnaise, vinegar, and black pepper in a small bowl until smooth. Drizzle this sauce over the chicken pieces in the rolls.

VEGETARIANS RECIPES

Pizza Portobello Mushrooms

Servings: 2   Cooking Time: 18 Minutes

Ingredients:

- 2 portobello mushroom caps, gills removed (see Figure 13-1)
- 1 teaspoon extra-virgin olive oil
- ¼ cup diced onion
- 1 teaspoon minced garlic
- 1 medium zucchini, shredded
- 1 teaspoon dried oregano
- ½ teaspoon black pepper
- ¼ teaspoon salt
- ⅓ cup marinara sauce
- ¼ cup shredded part-skim mozzarella cheese
- ¼ teaspoon red pepper flakes
- 2 tablespoons Parmesan cheese
- 2 tablespoons chopped basil

Directions:

1. Preheat the air fryer to 370°F.

2. Lightly spray the mushrooms with an olive oil mist and place into the air fryer to cook for 10 minutes, cap side up.

3. Add the olive oil to a pan and sauté the onion and garlic together for about 2 to 4 minutes. Stir in the zucchini, oregano, pepper, and salt, and continue to cook. When the zucchini has cooked down (usually about 4 to 6 minutes), add in the marinara sauce. Remove from the heat and stir in the mozzarella cheese.

4. Remove the mushrooms from the air fryer basket when cooking completes. Reset the temperature to 350°F.

5. Using a spoon, carefully stuff the mushrooms with the zucchini marinara mixture.

6. Return the stuffed mushrooms to the air fryer basket and cook for 5 to 8 minutes, or until the cheese is lightly browned. You should be able to easily insert a fork into the mushrooms when they're cooked.

7. Remove the mushrooms and sprinkle the red pepper flakes, Parmesan cheese, and fresh basil over the top.

8. Serve warm.

Falafel

Servings: 4   Cooking Time: 10 Minutes

Ingredients:

- 1 cup dried chickpeas
- ½ onion, chopped
- 1 clove garlic
- ¼ cup fresh parsley leaves
- 1 teaspoon salt
- ¼ teaspoon crushed red pepper flakes
- 1 teaspoon ground cumin
- ½ teaspoon ground coriander
- 1 to 2 tablespoons flour
- olive oil

- Tomato Salad
- 2 tomatoes, seeds removed and diced
- ½ cucumber, finely diced
- ¼ red onion, finely diced and rinsed with water
- 1 teaspoon red wine vinegar
- 1 tablespoon olive oil
- salt and freshly ground black pepper
- 2 tablespoons chopped fresh parsley

Directions:

1. Cover the chickpeas with water and let them soak overnight on the counter. Then drain the chickpeas and put them in a food processor, along with the onion, garlic, parsley, spices and 1 tablespoon of flour. Pulse in the food processor until the mixture has broken down into a coarse paste consistency. The mixture should hold together when you pinch it. Add more flour as needed, until you get this consistency.

2. Scoop portions of the mixture (about 2 tablespoons in size) and shape into balls. Place the balls on a plate and refrigerate for at least 30 minutes. You should have between 12 and 14 balls.

3. Preheat the air fryer to 380°F.

4. Spray the falafel balls with oil and place them in the air fryer. Air-fry for 10 minutes, rolling them over and spraying them with oil again halfway through the cooking time so that they cook and brown evenly.

5. Serve with pita bread, hummus, cucumbers, hot peppers, tomatoes or any other fillings you might like.

Roasted Vegetable Lasagna

Servings: 6   Cooking Time: 55 Minutes

Ingredients:

- 1 zucchini, sliced
- 1 yellow squash, sliced
- 8 ounces mushrooms, sliced
- 1 red bell pepper, cut into 2-inch strips
- 1 tablespoon olive oil
- 2 cups ricotta cheese
- 2 cups grated mozzarella cheese, divided
- 1 egg
- 1 teaspoon salt
- freshly ground black pepper
- ¼ cup shredded carrots

- ½ cup chopped fresh spinach
- 8 lasagna noodles, cooked
- Béchamel Sauce:
- 3 tablespoons butter
- 3 tablespoons flour
- 2½ cups milk
- ½ cup grated Parmesan cheese
- ½ teaspoon salt
- freshly ground black pepper
- pinch of ground nutmeg

Directions:

1. Preheat the air fryer to 400°F.

2. Toss the zucchini, yellow squash, mushrooms and red pepper in a large bowl with the olive oil and season with salt and pepper. Air-fry for 10 minutes, shaking the basket once or twice while the vegetables cook.

3. While the vegetables are cooking, make the béchamel sauce and cheese filling. Melt the butter in a medium saucepan over medium-high heat on the stovetop. Add the flour and whisk, cooking for a couple of minutes. Add the milk and whisk vigorously until smooth. Bring the mixture to a boil and simmer until the sauce thickens. Stir in the Parmesan cheese and season with the salt, pepper and nutmeg. Set the sauce aside.

4. Combine the ricotta cheese, 1¼ cups of the mozzarella cheese, egg, salt and pepper in a large bowl and stir until combined. Fold in the carrots and spinach.

5. When the vegetables have finished cooking, build the lasagna. Use a baking dish that is 6 inches in diameter and 4 inches high. Cover the bottom of the baking dish with a little béchamel sauce. Top with two lasagna noodles, cut to fit the dish and overlapping each other a little. Spoon a third of the ricotta cheese mixture and then a third of the roasted veggies on top of the noodles. Pour ½ cup of béchamel sauce on top and then repeat these layers two more times: noodles – cheese mixture – vegetables – béchamel sauce. Sprinkle the remaining mozzarella cheese over the top. Cover the dish with aluminum foil, tenting it loosely so the aluminum doesn't touch the cheese.

6. Lower the dish into the air fryer basket using an aluminum foil sling (fold a piece of aluminum foil into a strip about 2-inches wide by 24-inches long). Fold the ends of the aluminum foil over the top of the dish before returning the basket to the air fryer. Air-fry for 45 minutes, removing the foil for the last 2 minutes, to slightly brown the cheese on top.

7. Let the lasagna rest for at least 20 minutes to set up a little before slicing into it and serving.

Asparagus, Mushroom And Cheese Soufflés

Servings: 3   Cooking Time: 21 Minutes

Ingredients:

- butter
- grated Parmesan cheese
- 3 button mushrooms, thinly sliced
- 8 spears asparagus, sliced ½-inch long
- 1 teaspoon olive oil
- 1 tablespoon butter
- 4½ teaspoons flour
- pinch paprika
- pinch ground nutmeg
- salt and freshly ground black pepper
- ½ cup milk
- ½ cup grated Gruyère cheese or other Swiss cheese (about 2 ounces)
- 2 eggs, separated

Directions:

1. Butter three 6-ounce ramekins and dust with grated Parmesan cheese. (Butter the ramekins and then coat the butter with Parmesan by shaking it around in the ramekin and dumping out any excess.)

2. Preheat the air fryer to 400°F.

3. Toss the mushrooms and asparagus in a bowl with the olive oil. Transfer the vegetables to the air fryer and air-fry for 7 minutes, shaking the basket once or twice to redistribute the Ingredients while they cook.

4. While the vegetables are cooking, make the soufflé base. Melt the butter in a saucepan on the stovetop over medium heat. Add the flour, stir and cook for a minute or two. Add the paprika, nutmeg, salt and pepper. Whisk in the milk and bring the mixture to a simmer to thicken. Remove the pan from the heat and add the cheese, stirring to melt. Let the mixture cool for just a few minutes and then whisk the egg yolks in, one at a time. Stir in the cooked mushrooms and asparagus. Let this soufflé base cool.

5. In a separate bowl, whisk the egg whites to soft peak stage (the point at which the whites can almost stand up on the end of your whisk). Fold the whipped egg whites into the soufflé base, adding a little at a time.

6. Preheat the air fryer to 330°F.

7. Transfer the batter carefully to the buttered ramekins, leaving about ½-inch at the top. Place the ramekins into the air fryer basket and air-fry for 14 minutes. The soufflés should have risen nicely and be brown on top. Serve immediately.

Cheese Ravioli

Servings: 4

Cooking Time: 9 Minutes

Ingredients:

- 1 egg
- ¼ cup milk
- 1 cup breadcrumbs
- 2 teaspoons Italian seasoning
- ⅛ teaspoon ground rosemary
- ¼ teaspoon basil
- ¼ teaspoon parsley
- 9-ounce package uncooked cheese ravioli
- ¼ cup flour
- oil for misting or cooking spray

Directions:

1. Preheat air fryer to 390°F.
2. In a medium bowl, beat together egg and milk.
3. In a large plastic bag, mix together the breadcrumbs, Italian seasoning, rosemary, basil, and parsley.
4. Place all the ravioli and the flour in a bag or a bowl with a lid and shake to coat.
5. Working with a handful at a time, drop floured ravioli into egg wash. Remove ravioli, letting excess drip off, and place in bag with breadcrumbs.
6. When all ravioli are in the breadcrumbs' bag, shake well to coat all pieces.
7. Dump enough ravioli into air fryer basket to form one layer. Mist with oil or cooking spray. Dump the remaining ravioli on top of the first layer and mist with oil.
8. Cook for 5minutes. Shake well and spray with oil. Break apart any ravioli stuck together and spray any spots you missed the first time.
9. Cook 4 minutes longer, until ravioli puff up and are crispy golden brown.

Eggplant Parmesan

Servings: 4

Cooking Time: 8 Minutes Per Batch

Ingredients:

- 1 medium eggplant, 6–8 inches long
- salt
- 1 large egg
- 1 tablespoon water
- ⅔ cup panko breadcrumbs
- ⅓ cup grated Parmesan cheese, plus more for serving
- 1 tablespoon Italian seasoning
- ¾ teaspoon oregano
- oil for misting or cooking spray
- 1 24-ounce jar marinara sauce
- 8 ounces spaghetti, cooked
- pepper

Directions:

1. Preheat air fryer to 390°F.
2. Leaving peel intact, cut eggplant into 8 round slices about ¾-inch thick. Salt to taste.
3. Beat egg and water in a shallow dish.
4. In another shallow dish, combine panko, Parmesan, Italian seasoning, and oregano.
5. Dip eggplant slices in egg wash and then crumbs, pressing lightly to coat.
6. Mist slices with oil or cooking spray.
7. Place 4 eggplant slices in air fryer basket and cook for 8 minutes, until brown and crispy.
8. While eggplant is cooking, heat marinara sauce.
9. Repeat step 7 to cook remaining eggplant slices.
10. To serve, place cooked spaghetti on plates and top with marinara and eggplant slices. At the table, pass extra Parmesan cheese and freshly ground black pepper.

Quinoa Burgers With Feta Cheese And Dill

Servings: 6

Cooking Time: 10 Minutes

Ingredients:

- 1 cup quinoa (red, white or multi-colored)
- 1½ cups water
- 1 teaspoon salt
- freshly ground black pepper
- 1½ cups rolled oats
- 3 eggs, lightly beaten
- ¼ cup minced white onion
- ½ cup crumbled feta cheese
- ¼ cup chopped fresh dill
- salt and freshly ground black pepper
- vegetable or canola oil, in a spray bottle
- whole-wheat hamburger buns (or gluten-free hamburger buns*)
- arugula
- tomato, sliced
- red onion, sliced
- mayonnaise

Directions:

1. Make the quinoa: Rinse the quinoa in cold water in a saucepan, swirling it with your hand until any dry husks rise to the surface. Drain the quinoa as well as you can and then put the saucepan on the stovetop to dry and toast the quinoa. Turn the heat to medium-high and shake the pan regularly until you see the quinoa moving easily and can hear the seeds moving in the pan, indicating that they are dry. Add the water, salt and pepper. Bring the liquid to a boil and then reduce the heat to low or medium-low. You should see just a few bubbles, not a boil. Cover with a lid, leaving it askew and simmer for 20 minutes. Turn the heat off and fluff the quinoa with a fork. If there's any liquid left in the bottom of the pot, place it back on the burner for another 3 minutes or so. Spread the cooked quinoa out on a sheet pan to cool.

2. Combine the room temperature quinoa in a large bowl with the oats, eggs, onion, cheese and dill. Season with salt and pepper and mix well (remember that feta cheese is salty). Shape the mixture into 6 patties with flat sides (so they fit more easily into the air fryer). Add a little water or a few more rolled oats if necessary to get the mixture to be the right consistency to make patties.

3. Preheat the air-fryer to 400°F.

4. Spray both sides of the patties generously with oil and transfer them to the air fryer basket in one layer (you will probably have to cook these burgers in batches, depending on the size of your air fryer). Air-fry each batch at 400°F for 10 minutes, flipping the burgers over halfway through the cooking time.

5. Build your burger on the whole-wheat hamburger buns with arugula, tomato, red onion and mayonnaise.

Cheesy Enchilada Stuffed Baked Potatoes

Servings: 4   Cooking Time: 37 Minutes

Ingredients:

- 2 medium russet potatoes, washed
- One 15-ounce can mild red enchilada sauce
- One 15-ounce can low-sodium black beans, rinsed and drained
- 1 teaspoon taco seasoning
- ½ cup shredded cheddar cheese
- 1 medium avocado, halved
- ½ teaspoon garlic powder
- ¼ teaspoon black pepper
- ¼ teaspoon salt
- 2 teaspoons fresh lime juice
- 2 tablespoon chopped red onion
- ¼ cup chopped cilantro

Directions:

1. Preheat the air fryer to 390°F.

2. Puncture the outer surface of the potatoes with a fork.

3. Set the potatoes inside the air fryer basket and cook for 20 minutes, rotate, and cook another 10 minutes.

4. In a large bowl, mix the enchilada sauce, black beans, and taco seasoning.

5. When the potatoes have finished cooking, carefully remove them from the air fryer basket and let cool for 5 minutes.

6. Using a pair of tongs to hold the potato if it's still too hot to touch, slice the potato in half lengthwise. Use a spoon to scoop out the potato flesh and add it into the bowl with the enchilada sauce. Mash the potatoes with the enchilada sauce mixture, creating a uniform stuffing.

7. Place the potato skins into an air-fryer-safe pan and stuff the halves with the enchilada stuffing. Sprinkle the cheese over the top of each potato.

8. Set the air fryer temperature to 350°F, return the pan to the air fryer basket, and cook for another 5 to 7 minutes to heat the potatoes and melt the cheese.

9. While the potatoes are cooking, take the avocado and scoop out the flesh into a small bowl. Mash it with the back of a fork; then mix in the garlic powder, pepper, salt, lime juice, and onion. Set aside.

10. When the potatoes have finished cooking, remove the pan from the air fryer and place the potato halves on a plate. Top with avocado mash and fresh cilantro. Serve immediately.

Arancini With Marinara

Servings: 6

Cooking Time: 15 Minutes

Ingredients:

- 2 cups cooked rice
- 1 cup grated Parmesan cheese
- 1 egg, whisked
- ¼ teaspoon dried thyme
- ½ teaspoon dried oregano
- ½ teaspoon dried basil
- ½ teaspoon dried parsley
- 1 teaspoon salt
- ¼ teaspoon paprika
- 1 cup breadcrumbs
- 4 ounces mozzarella, cut into 24 cubes
- 2 cups marinara sauce

Directions:

1. In a large bowl, mix together the rice, Parmesan cheese, and egg.
2. In another bowl, mix together the thyme, oregano, basil, parsley, salt, paprika, and breadcrumbs.
3. Form 24 rice balls with the rice mixture. Use your thumb to make an indentation in the center and stuff 1 cube of mozzarella in the center of the rice; close the ball around the cheese.
4. Roll the rice balls in the seasoned breadcrumbs until all are coated.
5. Preheat the air fryer to 400°F.
6. Place the rice balls in the air fryer basket and coat with cooking spray. Cook for 8 minutes, shake the basket, and cook another 7 minutes.
7. Heat the marinara sauce in a saucepan until warm. Serve sauce as a dip for arancini.

Printed by Libri Plureos GmbH in Hamburg,
Germany